A C

THE POWER OF APPETITE CORRECTION

BERT HERRING, MD

www.BertHerring.com

OpKnox LLC

Jacksonville, Florida

www.opknox.com

P1.01.151009

ISBN-13 — 978-0692517376

ISBN-10 — 0692517375

LCCN — 2015913854

BOOK DESIGN AND ILLUSTRATIONS BY ALLISON HOLDRIDGE

CONTENTS

CONTENTS (CONTINUED)

Acknowledgments

Thank you to all of the Fast-5ers who have asked questions, described your experiences and shared your successes with others. My thanks also go out to the many physicians who have considered Fast-5 and found it a safe, effective plan worthy of sharing with their patients.

Bert Herring MD

Precautions

With the exception of a brief summary of practices that parents may choose to adopt for the benefit of their kids that begins on page 139, this guide is intended for adults. If you adopt any practice suggested for your appetite correction (AC) lifestyle, you accept the risk of choosing to do so.

If you are or may be pregnant or if you are nursing, consult your physician before adopting any practice suggested as part of an AC lifestyle.

Do not attempt to implement or maintain an AC lifestyle without a physician's supervision if you are taking any long-term medication or have a medical condition that is long-term in nature such as diabetes, epilepsy, heart disease, high blood pressure or if you've had a stroke. Obesity (greater than 20 percent overweight) is a long-term medical condition distinct from being overweight that involves substantial changes in physiologic status that may cause unpredictable responses to changes in meal content or schedule. If you are obese, please consult with and be monitored by a physician while starting and maintaining your AC lifestyle.

The material presented in this book is for your consideration and personal evaluation. It is not to be considered or acted on as medical advice.

Who is this book for?

This book is for the person who has surplus fat and wants to lose it; it is not intended to address the needs or interests of bodybuilders. Bodybuilders may use techniques similar to what is described in this book, but will likely be better served by looking to Martin Berkhan's leangains.com or Ori Hofmekler's *The Warrior Diet*. If you want to go from fat to lean, please read on.

measurement used to be bigger than my waist, and I'm afraid there's no going back. All I see now is fat, and I'm afraid there's no going back. All I see now is fat. I know it's true. I haven't been able to lose my muffin top! I don't want to shop in the plus-sized section. My ankles like mine. I used to have a waist. I want my pre-pregnancy body back. I had to keep buying bigger clothes. My inseam measurement used to be bigger than my waist. I passed 'big guy' status a long time ago. All I see no going back. My doctor said I'm killing myself. I know it's true. I haven't been able to lose my muffin top! My beer belly has to go! I don't want to shop in the plus-sized section. My kid asked me if cankles meant ankles like mine. I can't afford to keep buying my pre-pregnancy body back. I can't afford to keep buying measurement used to be bigger than my waist, and I'm afraid there's no going back. All I see now is fat, and I'm afraid there's no going back. I know it's true. I haven't been able to lose my muffin top. I don't want to shop in the plus-sized section. My kid asked me if the plus-sized section. My pre-preg

The Starting Line

It's been ten years since my first book, *The Fast-5 Diet and the Fast-5 Lifestyle*, was published. A Fast-5 lifestyle is simple. There is one rule: eat within five consecutive hours. That means you set a window of five hours, such as 1 pm to 6 pm or 5 pm to 10 pm and eat only within that window. During the five-hour window, you eat as you please, but you're not eating constantly for those five hours.

The simple Fast-5 lifestyle change has been working for thousands of people all around the world as a powerful and effective fat loss/weight maintenance tool. That adds up to thousands of years of user experience with Fast-5's schedule-restricted eating. The lessons learned from that experience plus new research findings and the introduction of a variety of other forms of intermittent fasting call for a fresh look at the subject. The Fast-5 schedule remains an excellent starting point for an appetite correction (AC) lifestyle. We'll talk more about AC later; let's start with some basics and ponder an important question.

What is the problem that a diet is supposed to fix?

2

If I asked you in person, the conversation might go something like this:

Me: "Why did you start reading this book?"
You: (looking at me funny) "Duh! Too much fat!"

It's more likely the conversation would avoid the three-letter F-word. It's a loaded word, so instead of "fat," your reply might be one of these typical answers:

"I haven't been able to lose my muffin top!"

"My beer belly has to go!"

"I don't want to shop in the plus-sized section."

"My kid asked me if cankles meant ankles like mine."

"I used to have a waist."

"I want my pre-pregnancy body back."

"I can't afford to keep buying bigger clothes."

"My inseam measurement used to be bigger than my waist."

"I passed 'big guy' status a long time ago. All I see now is fat, and I'm afraid there's no going back."

"My doctor said I'm killing myself. I know it's true."

Whatever it is that brings you here, it's clear that your surplus fat crossed a line and you decided to do something about it. It's important to note who decided it was time to do something about it. You decided! You decide when you have too much fat, and you decide how to manage the problem.

For now, though, it's time for us to get back to the f-word. I use it profusely throughout this book and fully accept that if this book is ever made into a movie, it will be rated R, so you may as well get used to it. Fat! Fat! Fat! There, I said it! Try saying the f-word out loud yourself: fat!

Surplus fat means more fat than you want or need. If you're like most people who are reading this book, you're looking for a diet to get rid of your surplus fat. Your goal is to be lean and healthy. It's obvious that by getting rid of the surplus fat, you'll reach that goal, right?

No, surplus fat is not the problem in need of correction. Surplus fat is a condition you'd like to correct. The underlying problem that needs to be fixed is the cause of the surplus fat. The cause and the condition are not the same thing. Correcting the condition (surplus fat) will not remove the cause. As long as the cause remains, even if you manage to correct the condition, the surplus fat will return.

For example, one way to remove surplus fat is by surgical liposuction. If a person with excess fat has some of it removed with liposuction, does

HOW IS IT DIFFERENT FROM WHERE YOU ARE NOW?

As you approach and achieve your goals, your goal body may change. Things you may have given up on years ago may suddenly become realistic goals, prompting you to adjust your goal body. What does your goal body look like? How does it feel to be running, dancing, playing and loving in your goal body?

THERE ARE TWO IMPORTANT THINGS TO TAKE FORWARD FROM THIS CHAPTER:

1. People with excess fat have not one but two problems to fix. There's a condition (having surplus fat, which can cause other problems) and there's a cause (overeating) that caused the condition.

2. You decided you had surplus fat. You decided to take action. You decide what your goal body looks like. You don't need numbers, tables or calculators to establish your goal or tell you when you've reached it. You know what your goal body looks like and feels like. If you don't know how your goal body would feel because you've been carrying surplus fat all your life,

you'll know when you get there. If you achieve your goal body and are encouraged to redefine your goal body to one that's even leaner, that's fine.

Here's some good news: there's one thing that can fix both the condition and the cause so you can achieve your goal body, and it doesn't require liposuckers, reality TV appearances or magic wands. It's the power of appetite correction (AC).

When you have read the rest of this book and put into practice the AC lifestyle that suits you best, you won't be following the ABC diet or the XYZ diet or Dr. Blah's diet or any other named diet—it won't even be a diet in the customary sense of the word. It will be your personal, customized AC lifestyle: a set of choices, habits and activities that works for you and works with your body rather than against it.

Writing down how your goal body looks and feels can make your goal feel more tangible.

I. LEARNING

Monetizing Misfortune

When we talk about the *root cause* of a problem, we're talking about the basic thing that's going wrong in the first place. Suppose the manager of a car production line notices cars are coming off the assembly line with cracked windshields. If the manager adds workers to the assembly line to replace the windshields, the windshields are repaired and the cars are sent to the dealers in perfect condition. That's symptomatic treatment: the manager is fixing the condition without addressing its cause. That's not very smart, is it? The manager's fix adds costs and has to be maintained indefinitely to deliver cars without defects, and it doesn't fix the problem. On the other hand, it does create jobs for windshield fixers, and the windshield makers are happy to sell more windshields.

A good manager would find the cause of the problem by investigating what's cracking the windshields in the first place. Maybe a robot's sensor is broken, allowing the robot's arm to swing against the windshield and crack it. If the manager fixes the robot, the problem is eliminated for the long term and there is no need to add workers to the assembly line to replace the windshields. With the cause fixed, only the windshields that came off the line cracked have to be fixed. When that's done, the manager has addressed both the condition (cracked windshields) and the cause: bad robot (no relation to J.J. Abrams).

The manager identified the cause and repaired the robot, but can still look even further to identify a root cause—the reason the robot broke. The manager determines that proper maintenance on the robot was done, but a part of the robot was faulty. The manager switches suppliers for that part to a source with better quality control. By doing so, the manager addresses the root cause. Now, not only is the windshield problem resolved and the robot fixed, but the same problem is not likely to happen again because the root cause has been identified and corrected.

How does this approach work in the case of surplus fat? Many people employ a variety of techniques to manage surplus fat, including dieting, drugs, surgery, shapewear, vertical stripes or running on treadmills just to burn off excess calorie intake. These techniques may, for some, successfully prevent, remove or hide surplus fat, but at what cost?

Take a moment to consider this: How much sense does it make to spend money for access to a treadmill so we can run miles just to burn off calories that we also paid for in the form of food? Wouldn't it be better to cut out the excess food intake, and with it, cut the need for treadmill mileage? Why don't we just stop eating excess food?

Let's consider how we follow the lead of advertisers, who create a relentless stream of advertisements created to persuade us to buy and consume food. They're monetizing human vulnerability, but it goes deeper. The advertising is also trying to persuade us to buy drugs, treadmills, surgery and shapewear so that we can fix or hide our surplus fat problem without addressing the root cause. The sad truth is that by offering solutions that fail to address the root cause of the problem, the healthcare/fitness industry is monetizing our misfortune.

What if it were possible to address the root cause of surplus fat and eliminate the need for dieting, drugs and all the pseudo-solutions?

Let's return to our assembly line analogy and look at what's producing the condition of surplus fat and what's supporting the industry built around addressing the condition without getting rid of the root cause.

GOING STEP-BY-STEP UP THE ASSEMBLY LINE OF SURPLUS FAT:

Step 1. The surplus fat itself: The fat stores become excessive because food absorbed from the gut after eating is not needed for fuel by other tissues. The fat cells store the excess fuel just like they're supposed to. No problem here! The fat cells are doing what they're told and working like they should.

Step 2. Too much fat storage is caused by too much food entering the gut, and that comes from overeating. If a person would just choose to eat less, the problem would go away. Does that mean that addressing the root cause is simply a matter of people making better choices?

Is the overeating person's willpower faulty? No.

Step 3. To find the root cause, we have to look at why we eat more than we need when we're already burdened by excess fat. Do we want to add to the excess? No! While many individuals with surplus fat have come to terms with the condition, accept it and deal with it, there are few who would decline to flip a switch, if doing so would take them from fat to lean without an ongoing battle of willpower.

People encumbered by surplus fat know they eat more than their body needs. They fight to eat less every day and the outcome of the battle is clear: they lose the battle and gain fat. They keep overeating. A person with surplus fat knows that eating less can bring very valuable rewards: better health, more social acceptance, an enhanced sense of well-being, less stereotyping and more. Even with these great incentives, they don't exercise their willpower and make the choice that gets rid of their excess fat.

Have you ever found yourself eating when you were not even hungry? You ate despite knowing you did not need food, and you truly want a lean body much more than you wanted whatever food you were eating at the moment. Why did you choose to eat rather than make progress toward a leaner body? Was it just a failure of willpower? Are you just weak-minded? No!

There's a lot more to the overeating problem than willpower.

Two issues are tangled together in our search for the root cause of overeating:

1. Why does your preference to eat less fail to keep you from eating?

2. What is it that you're fighting when you lose this willpower battle?

We'll pull the tangle apart and look at both aspects, but first we have to consider something called infoclutter.

pounds or mo... natural! Minimally invasive su... n seconds! 24-hour miracle diet! All natural cleanse! ... natural all in one formula! Control your appetite with del... roved! Smooth, creamy and delicious! Miraculous weight ... x weight loss medications prescribed by our doctors! Tri... Miracle diet and detox supplement! Pay a few bucks, feel ... rough ingredients as seen on TV! 10 pounds in 10 minutes! ose 15 pounds or more! Lose 3x more weight than dieting ... ods! 100% natural! Minimally invasive surgery options! ... pack in seconds! 24-hour miracle diet! All natural cleans... nent! Natural all in one formula! Control your appetite w... and improved! Smooth, creamy and delicious! Miraculous ... stom Rx weight loss medications prescribed by our docto... Miracle diet and detox supplement! Pay a few bucks... seen on TV! 10 pounds in 10 ... ...weight than ...

I. LEARNING

Infoclutter

This likely isn't your first time at the diet rodeo, and you may be wondering why it's so hard to succeed. It's just a matter of eating less and exercising more, right? You see lots of stories in the various media channels about miraculous fat loss. Is it like the lottery? Some people win and others don't? Random chance? Why are others experiencing "miraculous" fat loss and you can't do the same?

Those fat loss stories make it past the editor's desk because they're rare and they cultivate interest and sales. If 100-pound fat loss happened routinely, it wouldn't seem miraculous and the stories wouldn't be of interest. One of the reasons it's so hard to lose fat is that in the fat-loss tug-of-war, the power is on the opposite end of the rope from you. That means a lot of what you hear is infoclutter from those pulling against you—stuff that sounds good, and may have some real facts in it, but doesn't really help solve the problem. Who wins the tug-of-war if you eat too much? As the saying goes, follow the money:

- Food producers and sellers

- Drug and supplement makers and sellers

- Clothing and shapewear makers and sellers

- Manufacturers and sellers of fitness equipment, apps and devices

- Fitness center owners and staff

- Medical center owners and staff

- Weight loss counseling and packaged meal services

- Fraudulent shysters and shameless purveyors of ineffective supplements
- Supermarket tabloids offering ways to "Lose 23 Pounds!"
- Manufacturers and sellers of enabling devices: electric scooter chairs, wide-bottom toilet seats, etc.
- Diet book authors, publishers and sellers (yes, that includes me.)

NOW, HERE'S A LIST OF THOSE WHO STAND TO BENEFIT FROM YOU EATING LESS:

- You (you'll feel better and probably either spend less on food or spend as much, but enhance the quality)
- Your family (because you'll be happier and will probably live longer)
- Your insurance company
- Your employer, if any, because you'll likely be more productive and have fewer sick days when you feel good, and your employer may get a "healthy workplace" discount on insurance if most employees are lean and don't smoke
- Me (because I enjoy seeing people succeed in their efforts to lose fat, and also because someone might ask how you did it, which might prompt them to buy this book. For both meaning and monetary reasons, I'm rooting for your success!)

You, your family, your employer, your insurance company and me on the same team? It may seem unlikely, but it's true! If you look at the list of those who benefit from you gaining fat and staying fat, it's easy to see why there's a lot of interest in helping you get rid of some fat, but not much interest in your success or addressing the root cause. If you were able to address the root cause and the condition on your own, you wouldn't need anything from anyone in the first list!

It's time to be an outlaw. It's time to be a desperado and hold up the gravy train delivering money to everyone on the follow-the-money list.

An appetite correcting lifestyle gives you license to break the following rules:

- Clean your plate.
- Breakfast is the most important meal of the day.
- Don't eat late at night.
- Eat every few hours to keep your metabolism revved.
- Eat only low fat foods.
- Don't swim immediately after eating.
- Don't play with your food.
- If you don't eat your meat, you can't have any pudding.

Desperados make their own rules, so take liberties and make modifications:

- Eat ~~all your~~ veggies.
- ~~Don't~~ play! ~~with your food.~~

Here's one rule that's a keeper, even for desperados:

- Avoid trans fats.

To address the root cause of surplus fat, we have to look a little deeper into what's going on. . .

I. LEARNING

Appetite vs. Hunger

There's an autopilot in your brain's core. You've probably heard that your body has an automatic "fight or flight" response. The nerve network driving the fight-or-flight response is called the sympathetic nervous system. There's also a balancing network called the parasympathetic nervous system, which is nicknamed the "feed-or-breed" system because of its importance in regulating digestion as well as controlling reproductive activities from arousal to labor. Together, the sympathetic and parasympathetic nerve networks make up the autonomic nervous system. The fight-or-flight and feed-or-breed nicknames are helpful but incomplete, since the automatic functions our bodies handle go far beyond fighting, fleeing, feeding and breeding.

Do you tell your heart to beat faster when you exercise? Do you have to remind yourself to breathe? No, your autonomic system takes care of those things for you, even while you're sleeping. The breathing center and heart rate control center are built into your brain's primitive core. This primitive core is very similar to the same part of the brain in non-human animals.

Warm-blooded animals from a tiny two-gram hummingbird to a 190 metric ton blue whale have to regulate their breathing and heart rate too, so they have a similar automatic system in their brain's core. When you look at all the things your body does, it's a good thing many of them are automatic systems. Imagine what it would be like if you had to think about digesting your food, or if you had to coordinate muscle movements in your gut and airway so that when you vomit, you don't barf stomach acid into your lungs. What if you had to decide when and how much to sweat to keep your body cool when you're running on a hot summer day? Automatic systems control a lot of things without us even thinking about them. There's little doubt we'd screw things up badly if we had to think about all of the things our automatic systems control! Suppose you had to consciously tell your heart to beat every second and three seconds without a beat meant you'd fall unconscious and die. How long would you live? Even if you could somehow make it through the day, you'd die as soon as you fell asleep. Your body handles these housekeeping details all at the same time. Imagine a woman in a delivery room about to have a baby: her automatic systems adjust her visual focus and pupil size while maintaining her heart rate, blood pressure and breathing rate, digesting her dinner and filtering her blood, all while she's sweating, grimacing and delivering a baby. Even with all that going on, if she happens to vomit, her automatic systems will coordinate the process so her lungs are protected from inhaling stomach acid.

Want to see your autopilot at work? How long can you suppress your drive to breathe? Most people can manage a minute or two at best before the breathing center kicks in, vetoes the silliness coming from the conscious part of the brain and forces a breath. If it didn't, a person could commit suicide just by breath-holding. Have you ever heard of anyone doing that? It doesn't happen. The autonomic system takes control away from the conscious mind when survival is at stake. The brain-core autopilot steps in and keeps us from killing ourselves by choosing not to breathe or forgetting to do so.

In addition to controlling your heart rate and breathing, the primitive brain core also controls other things. It controlled your growth as you grew from a baby to an adult, and it controlled your sexual maturation. It demands that you sleep, but monitors sounds and will awaken you from sleep if something unusual happens. It controls your temperature and determines whether you need to sweat or not to cool off, and it controls your sexual cycles, urges and responses.

HERE'S A SHORT LIST OF SOME THINGS YOUR BODY CONTROLS AUTOMATICALLY:

- Sleep
- Pupil diameter
- Eye focus distance
- Balance
- Growth
- Sexual maturation
- Coordination of walking
- Digestion (progression through gut and secretion of digestive enzymes)
- Vomiting
- Sneezing
- Flinching
- Startle response

- Breathing rate
- Heart rate
- Blood pressure
- Arousal and orgasm
- Pulse
- Sweating
- Crying
- Coughing
- Salivation (mouth watering)
- Labor & Delivery
- Lactation (letdown)
- Urination (peeing)

· ·

You've seen some of what your body does automatically, so now we will look at another automatic function of your body's brain-core autopilot system: appetite.

APPETITE

Appetite is the drive to eat, which is generated by the appetite center of the brain. Appetite is one of the many functions maintained by the body's autopilot system. The part of the brain that controls appetite sits in the core of the brain alongside other basic functions that are essential for life. Appetite is as primitive and controlling a drive as the urge to breathe, sleep or have sex. You have about as much control of your appetite as you do your temperature or your heart rate. Appetite is not the same as somatic hunger, which is a sensation you feel in your belly, or limbic hunger, which is the drive to continue eating until full once you start eating. Because it's part of the primitive core of the brain, the human appetite center is very similar to the appetite centers of other warm-blooded animals.

Look around and you'll see the appetite center working as perfectly as your breathing center does. Look at all the animals in the world not fed by humans. Have you seen any wild birds that are so fat they cannot fly? Have you ever seen an obese lion, tiger, wolf or chimpanzee? Don't they all look like they're at their ideal body size? Animals hunt or forage only when they need to. Animal appetite centers keep their bodies stocked with some fat reserve, but not so much they're obese. Non-human animals do no calorie counting, use no apps, food logs or drugs, yet they eat precisely enough to have some fat in reserve, but not so much that they grow fat and become easy prey for other animals. The ability of an animal's appetite center to push up the drive to eat when fat stores are low and drop it when fat stores are abundant resembles a thermostat, so the appetite center is often called the appestat.

Earlier we saw that there are two intertwined problems: (1) the drive to eat overwhelms conscious choice to the contrary and (2) the human drive to overeat persists in spite of the presence of surplus fat. Here's the explanation behind the first problem.

WHY THE APPESTAT WINS

Sigmund Freud observed that the conscious mind is like a jockey sitting on a horse (the autopilot brain core) that has a strong will of its own. When the appestat in the core of your brain determines that you need to eat, you will eat unless the drive is overridden by another brain-core system such as fight-or-flight. The appestat can set eating behavior in motion against your will—that's appetite driven eating (ADE). It's no different than when your brain core takes control of your body under many other circumstances. If you watch a scary movie and you know something is about to startle you, you can try to make yourself stay calm. Dahhh-dum . . . dahhhhh-dum. The music stirs up anticipation. Dahhhh-dum . . . dahhhh-dum. You know something is about to happen. Dahhh-dum. . .dahhh-dum! You steel yourself. You feel your heart racing. Dah-dum-dah-dum-dah-dum! You expect the unexpected. Dah-dum-dah-dum-dah-dum! The monster/villain/shark attacks! You jump! Even though you know you're completely safe in the theater or your living room, your brain-core fight-or-flight response takes control, makes you jump and sends your heart racing faster. You may even feel it now, just thinking about it.

The same thing happens when you try to hold your breath for a long time. Eventually, the brain core wrestles control of your behavior from your conscious mind (which resides mostly in the outer layer of your brain, the cortex) and makes you breathe. There are some circumstances, such as hunger strikes, when people have been able to override the appestat, but these are rare and involve not eating at all rather than choosing to eat less. By avoiding eating entirely, a hunger striker keeps the appestat from having the opportunity to take control of eating behavior.

You and your brain are built to survive whimsical notions like choosing not to breathe or forgetting to eat. The appestat initiates eating behavior and overrides the objections coming from the cortex. The result of this core-driven behavior may be familiar to you. If you've ever been eating while recognizing you're not even hungry, you've seen your appestat run over your cortex's petty objections, controlling your behavior with its survival-mode power.

Now we're getting somewhere in our search for a root cause. We can see appestat-driven eating behaviors emerge from the brain core and override conscious preferences. That explains why willpower loses the battle to eat less almost all the time. However, it doesn't explain why the appestat is forcing you to eat more when there's already plenty of fat stored.

The prevalence of people encumbered by surplus fat makes it obvious that something's wrong, and it's not just you. Something is confusing a lot of appestats, because appetite is clearly driving people to eat when they don't need to. The appestat is either not getting good information about how much fat is stored, or it's getting that information but miscalculating the need for more food intake.

captivity are ...

...mals that graze tend to do so on ...

...ent density. Other animals must hunt, gather or fight f...

...ating and acquiring food. Other animals must tear, bite, gna...

...h no tools, slowing eating and digestion. Other animals rar...

...o matter what the occasion may be. Other animals eat no s...

...and most eat very little starch. Other animals' use of salt

...ings, fragrances and flavor enhancers has not been reporte...

...rds, mammals, reptiles, amphibians, fish and bugs, eat bugs...

...y spend energy cooling or heating their bodies. Other anim...

...night cycle with seasonal variation and display little inter...

...ing alarms. Other animals don't have fixed schedules, but ...

...hythm. Animals eating on schedules in captivity are at risk...

...als don't eat cooked food. Other animals that graze tend to ...

...es, which have low nutrient density. Other animals r...

...locating and acquiring food. Oth...

...ing eating a...

Humans vs. Other Animals

If we accept that the mammalian appetite center works in nature, and the human appetite center is similar to other mammals, then something must be confusing the human appetite center. What could be causing the confusion? Let's compare the obvious differences between the way people eat and the way other animals eat:

SCHEDULE

- Humans eat on a schedule whether hungry or not, many times per day; food is often presented/consumed regardless of hunger.

- Other animals don't have fixed schedules, but may eat on a loose daily rhythm. Animals eating on schedules in captivity (pets and zoo animals) are at risk for overfeeding and may become obese.

PACKAGING

- Humans package, cook or modify most foods.

- Other animals don't eat cooked food, except for buzzards eating roadkill off the shimmering summertime blacktop.

GRAZING

- Humans may eat throughout the day, grazing on nutrient-dense foods like fruit, seeds and sugary snacks.

- Other animals that graze tend to do so on foods such as grass and leaves, which have low nutrient density.

ACCESS

- Humans have easy access to food; very little energy is spent acquiring food.
- Other animals must hunt, gather or fight for food. Most activity involves locating and acquiring food.

PRE-DIGESTION

- Humans cut, chop, purée and make julienne fries out of food using tools, and grind some foods such as wheat and peanuts to fine powder, predigesting the food so little or no chewing is required; consumption and digestion are fast and absorption of calories is complete.
- Other animals must tear, bite, gnaw and chew raw foods with no tools, slowing eating and digestion.

FOOD COMPOSITION

- Humans consume a large proportion of calorie intake in the form of simple sugars and cooked starches, which are quickly converted to sugars during digestion.
- Other animals eat no sugar or very little sugar, and most eat very little starch. Those eating sugars tend to be very active (hummingbirds) or eat sugars only occasionally (bears).

FLAVOR ENHANCEMENT

- Humans add salt, preservatives, flavorings, fragrances and other enhancers to food.
- Other animals' use of flavor enhancers, salt shakers, flavorings, fragrances and preservatives has not been reported.

SOCIAL/PEER PRESSURE

- Humans encourage others to eat in most social situations.
- Other animals rarely encourage others to eat no matter what the occasion may be.

FOOD SCIENCE & ENGINEERING

- Humans engineer foods to be especially attractive/addictive to other humans.
- Other animals seldom apply to work as food scientists.

BUGS

- Humans rarely eat bugs.
- Other animals, such as birds, mammals, reptiles, amphibians, fish and bugs, eat bugs.

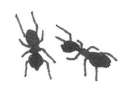 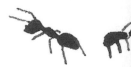

ENVIRONMENT

- Humans eat and live in environmentally controlled surroundings, rarely sweating or shivering.

- Other animals frequently spend energy cooling or heating their bodies, such as panting, shivering or activating brown (heat-generating) fat.

HYDRATION

- Humans often sip beverages such as coffee, tea, water and sodas throughout the day.

- Other animals do not purchase 30+ ounce lattes or 32-ounce portions of sugar water (a.k.a. soft drinks and sports drinks). Water sources are associated with hazards such as alligators, piranhas, crocodiles, snakes and parasites that may consume the drinker or parts thereof.

SCHEDULE

- Humans live on a schedule dictated by work, school and clocks; electric lighting is used to replace sunlight and extend active hours.

- Other animals thrive on a sun-based day/night cycle with seasonal variation and display little interest in acquiring clocks or setting alarms.

ACTIVITY

- Humans are relatively sedentary in most jobs, with an increasing amount of low-activity "screen time" watching screens for work, play, communication and entertainment.

- Other animals must participate in finding and consuming food as the primary job, and success at this role is a prerequisite for participation in other jobs such as mating and protecting self and offspring. Sedentary approaches to this primary task are rare among warm-blooded animals but are common among clams, oysters, sponges and anemones.

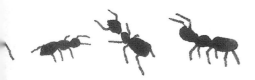

out half of a black-and-white s
20 calories = a bite of a hot dog. 20 calories
calories = one peppermint hard candy. 20 calories = tw
bout two sips of cola. 20 calories = five pieces of colorfu
your mouth, not in your hand. 20 calories = about half o
= about half of a black-and-white sandwich cookie. 20 ca
ips. 20 calories = a bite of a hot dog. 20 calories = one b
ar. 20 calories = one peppermint hard candy. 20 calories
s = about two sips of cola. 20 calories = five pieces of col
lt in your mouth, not in your hand. 20 calories = about ha
ries = about half of a black-and-white sandwich cookie. 20
o chips. 20 calories = a bite of a hot dog. 20 calories = o
dy bar. 20 calories = one peppermint hard candy. 20 calo
about two sips of cola. 20 calories = five pieces of
in your hand. 20 calories = abou
dwich cook

I. LEARNING

The Key Differences

This list of differences could go on and on. Is it clear which of the items from the list in the last chapter is the culprit that's confusing human appetite centers? It's not, but we can be pretty sure that an absence of bugs in our diet is not a big deal.

Our appestats deserve some credit for doing as well as they do under the circumstances. Even though they may be a bit confused, our appestats aren't off by much. The average American gains about two pounds per year, which corresponds to an annual calorie excess of about 7,000 calories. That may sound like a lot, but it means the typical fat-gainer has an average daily surplus of only 20 calories. That's only 1.3 percent of a 1,500 calorie per day diet, which means it's still 98.7 percent accurate—an A+! Twenty calories is less than half of a popular brand's black-and-white sandwich cookie! Twenty calories is just a couple of potato chips too much every day!

If your appestat were really messed up—say just ten percent out of whack on the upside—you'd double your weight every eight years. If it were ten percent too low, you'd starve within five years. Your appestat isn't broken; it's just slightly out of tune.

The root cause of human appetite confusion probably includes more than one item on the list of differences in the previous chapter as well as one or more items that are not on the list. We could ditch our electric lights, turn off the heaters, air conditioners, televisions, computers and blenders, stop buying packaged flour and pasta, start eating bugs and start growing all of our own food and eating it all raw and unprocessed and see what happens, but most people aren't too keen on doing that.

It feels good to know exactly what's going on, but in the case of the out-of-tune appestat, not knowing the exact root cause doesn't mean we can't solve our problem. Figuring out where the problem is and where it's not is a big step forward. It allows us to stop wasting time and energy problem-solving in the wrong place and guides us toward the discovery and implementation of sustainable solutions. Until our scientific discoveries catch up to explain our real-life experiences and observations, we can simply embrace the mystery and respect it with character, an approach that's served many successful problem solvers well over the years.

Gremlins have been blamed for things going wrong in all sorts of vehicles since the 1940s, especially things that had no clear explanation. Let's blame appetite confusion on gremlins—sneaky masters of appetite confusion that insist on messing with the appetite center in your primary vehicle: your body. As long as we can find some tools to keep the gremlins from confusing your appetite center, we don't have to know exactly how they're confusing it. Knowing one's body-vehicle well is the first step in keeping the gremlins from messing with it, so we'll get to that next.

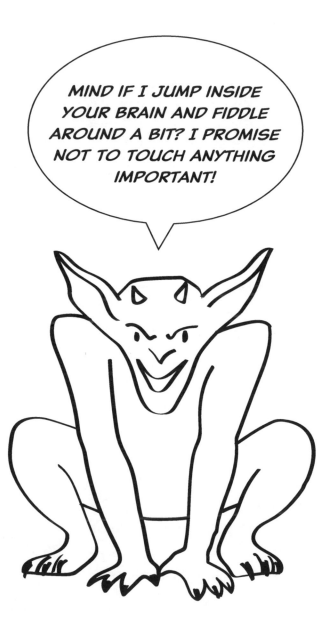

I. LEARNING

Terms

FAT

Fat is not a demon. You may not think so, but fat is a wonderful thing. It's essential for life, and it's a major organ of the human body. Your body, including your brain, needs quite a bit of fat just to work normally. Fat is essential for building cells. Having some reserve fat is both a good thing and a natural feature that has allowed individuals of our species to survive weeks to months with little or no food. Acting as nature's refrigerator, fat allows us to store fuel in times of plenty. Once fat is stored, it's automatically protected from rot, bugs and other critters and it won't go bad during a power failure. Fat is also good to have if you've just fallen into extremely cold water because fat is a good insulator. A thick layer of fat under the skin of whales, walruses and seals allows them to keep their body core warm in Arctic temperatures with no need for parkas or earmuffs.

It's the surplus of fat that causes health, social and job troubles, so remember fat is good stuff—it's just the surplus of fat that's troublesome.

What is fat? As mentioned before, fat is fuel. The fat from whale blubber was once a common source of fuel for lamps—clear evidence that fat is stored energy. A lamp burning fat releases that stored energy as heat and light. Fat is such a good way to store energy that some vehicles can run on vegetable oil, which is a kind of fat. Vegetable fat (oil) is used instead of animal fat because vegetable oil is cheaper and tends to be liquid at lower temperatures, while animal fats (such as butter or lard) are usually solid at room temperature. As you can imagine, it's more difficult to pump solid animal fat than liquid vegetable fat into an engine's cylinders as fuel. Solid animal fat (tallow) was also once widely used to make candles, just as wax is used today. Human fat is largely the same as any other animal's fat, so as gross as it may sound, liposuctioned fat from people could be used to power engines, candles or lamps. And no, even with epidemic obesity, we're not going to reach energy independence that way.

A car engine running on fat (or any other fuel) produces mechanical energy and heat, just as your muscles do. The underlying chemical process of fat combustion, which combines oxygen with fuel to release energy, is the same for oil lamps, candles, engines and your body.

Fat is just one of the fuels that the tiny flexible-fuel engines called mitochondria (my-tuh-kon-dree-uh) that power the cells of your body can use. Mitochondria can also run on bits of sugars like glucose or fructose, or on alcohol or ketones, which we'll talk about later.

Although extra fat may be good in some special circumstances like falling overboard in the Arctic Ocean or washing up on a deserted island, surplus fat is generally an undesirable condition: it increases the risk of nine of the top ten causes of death. It probably comes as no surprise to you that surplus fat can be a severe social and employment obstacle as well as a health encumbrance.

FAT VS. WEIGHT

Fat, then, is very good stuff to have around, as long as there's not too much of it. In medical terms, having too much fat could be called "adipomegaly," but the more convenient term "overweight" is usually used instead. Fat is not the only thing that influences body weight, and keeping attention only on body weight can be misleading, because a person's weight can quickly change up or down a pound or two even though there's been no change in the total amount of fat. Using the term "surplus fat" also reminds us that having some fat is essential for good health. It's not a question of fat vs. non-fat—it's whether you have enough or too much. How you refer to the surplus fat—obesity, overweight, adipomegaly, overfat, fat or fluffy—doesn't matter as long as you manage the root cause, the problem causing the condition.

DIET VS. LIFESTYLE

In its most common usage, the word "diet" usually means a way of eating that one follows for a few months to lose fat. In this book and in the general scientific sense, a diet isn't just eating to lose weight—your diet is whatever you're eating. It's not what you plan to eat, but what you really eat. Everyone has a diet unless they're on a long-term fast, and that fast is going to end—one way or another.

It's time to stop thinking about diets as a temporary thing, because temporary fixes just can't last. Once the diet is done, the dieter resumes the same way of eating that caused the fat gain, with a predictable outcome: the fat lost through dieting is regained. Many people have a long history of successful dieting efforts that they have alternated with their traditional way of eating, which is the way of eating that made them fat in the first place. Because the usual way of eating reliably causes fat gain, alternating that with a series of temporary diets leads to a yo-yo pattern of loss followed by gain. It's important to remember that the problem here is not the down side of the yo-yo—that part works! The problem is the up side—the fat that was lost returns when the traditional way of eating is resumed. It's remarkable that the traditional three meals a day (3MAD) way of eating, the way that's supposedly healthy, is contributing to the largest, most costly health problem that so-called developed countries have ever seen. How did that happen?

3MAD

If the down (diet) side of the yo-yo is doing its job, why does the dieter's fat keep returning after resuming the usual diet? Clearly there's something amiss with that "normal" diet! Remember the two-pound-per-year average gain we talked about earlier? Typical Americans who gain that much are most often doing so on a 3MAD schedule, which they maintain because they believe that to be the healthy choice, despite evidence to the contrary accumulating on their own bodies.

While relentless fat gain may be a common outcome for humans in Western cultures, that doesn't mean it's normal, and it's certainly not best for health. The 3MAD schedule started as an attempt by common folks to emulate rich people who had no better way to indulge themselves and demonstrate their wealth than eating frequently. In the early 20th century, advertisers—particularly breakfast cereal companies—started pushing consumption to increase profits. The trend toward ever-greater consumption continues today as advertisers encourage a fourth meal and encourage kids to snack between meals. Schools and parents offering frequent snacks and juice have become unknowing accomplices contributing to child obesity. The 3MAD schedule is a contrast to ancient Rome, where one who ate more than one meal a day was deemed a glutton. 3MAD was not created as a scientifically-tested optimal eating schedule for humans—it was created through a vicious cycle of advertising, profits, habits and ignorance that has helped spawn an obesity-generating culture. 3MAD may be troublesome on its own, but how often is it really just 3MAD? Isn't 3MAD often 3MAD "plus" (3MAD+) with the "plus" being a snack here and there, maybe a morning snack and an afternoon snack as many schools are teaching children, plus a bit of candy, okay, well maybe two bits of candy, no make that three bits. All right, four bits of candy, no more... well, five's kind of a nice, round number, we'll stop there with a soda to wash it down. Now, don't we have some chips somewhere?

FASTING

Fasting means going without food for some time, but fasting has no specific duration attached to it. Most people eating on a customary schedule of three meals a day have a dinner-to-breakfast fasting span of about 12 hours, so a 12-hour interval between meals is very common and would not generally be considered fasting. There are beneficial changes that occur with fasting, so the best definition of what length of time constitutes fasting might be "as long as it takes for at least one of the beneficial changes associated with fasting to occur." Those fasting-associated changes are subtle and vary in their onset from person to person, so determining how long one must go without food to reach the point of benefit can be very difficult. For now, it's practical to regard fasting as going without food for at least 50 percent longer than the longest interval between meals on a customary (3MAD) schedule: 12 hours x 1.5 = 18 hours. A better definition of fasting—one defined by changes that occur in the body as a result of fasting—may come along in the next few years as we learn more about the beneficial changes that occur as a result of fasting.

There are countless variations and subtleties in the ways that religious and philosophical practitioners define fasting. Religious fasting is often dependent on sunrise and sunset, which vary with the season and latitude, so these descriptions of fasting will not align with a fixed duration or other scientific definition.

NOT SO FAST!

"Juice fasting" isn't fasting at all. It's a liquid diet. While the inconvenience of turning all your food into liquid before consuming it may be sufficient to reduce intake, it's not fasting. Once food passes from your stomach to your intestine, it's almost all juice anyway—your teeth and the churning acid of your stomach do the juicing. A juice diet isn't sustainable for most people, and a diet you can't maintain indefinitely isn't worth starting. So please—if you're going to consume only juice, call it what it is: a juice diet or juicing—it's not fasting.

INTERMITTENT FASTING

Intermittent fasting (IF) is any repeating schedule of fasting alternating with periods of eating, where the fasting period fits the description above. "Intermittent" sometimes means sporadic or unreliable, but in this case, intermittent means that fasting stops and starts on a defined schedule.

METABOLISM

Chemicals are often thought of as unnatural or artificial, but chemicals are the basic components of everything in nature, including our bodies. Water is one chemical; salt is another. Glucose (blood sugar), insulin, fat and oxygen are all chemicals, too. Your metabolism is the collection of all the chemical reactions going on between all the chemicals in your body, such as combining fat with oxygen. This collection of millions of chemical reactions we call metabolism is going on all the time as long as you're alive. As was mentioned earlier, the fat-plus-oxygen chemical reaction that occurs in your body is the same chemical reaction that's going on when you burn a tallow candle or light an oil lamp. Instead of giving off heat and light as a candle or lamp does, your body captures the energy released by the chemical reaction. Your body uses the captured energy to move your muscles and build or repair your body parts. Without energy, your cells don't just sit there like a flashlight with a dead battery; they die. When too many of your cells die to keep your systems working, you die. To burn fuel for energy, you must have fuel and oxygen. To get oxygen, you must breathe. To get fuel, you must eat or draw from your body's stored fuel, almost all of which is fat. Your body, via the autopilot in your brain core, makes sure your body gets both fuel and oxygen to maintain the energy flow needed to support the constant buzz of the millions of chemical reactions that make up your metabolism.

Fat burning is just one of the millions of amazingly complex chemical reactions going on in the human body. Without the chemicals comprising our bodies and the constant process of changing them to different chemicals through chemical reactions, we would not be alive. Poisons are chemicals that interfere with one or more of the chemical reactions of metabolism, and if the interference is bad enough, the chemical reactions stop, the cells die and the body dies. Metabolism, the set of millions of ongoing chemical reactions that support the body's functions, is what a living person has that a dead body does not have: life!

METABOLIC RATE

The amount of energy needed each day to keep all those life-sustaining chemical reactions going and make it possible for our bodies to do the things we want them to do is called the metabolic rate. The metabolic rate is frequently called metabolism, as in "I have a low metabolism" or "boost your metabolism," but there's a difference. Metabolism is what's happening, and the metabolic rate is how fast it's happening. The basal metabolic rate (BMR) measures how much fuel your body needs every day just to stay alive with no activity at all.

The metabolic rate is not a measure of how much work the body's little cellular engines can do, like saying "a 250 horsepower engine" or "a 15 kilowatt generator," but a measure of how busy the cellular engines are as they go about doing what they do. The metabolic rate is similar to a tachometer, which shows how fast an engine is running. Seeing the true metabolic rate of a car's engine would require a gauge not seen on many cars: fuel flow. An inefficient, poorly tuned small engine can slurp up more fuel in the same amount of time as a more efficient, more powerful engine. If the two engines have the same fuel flow, they have the same metabolic rate. The same is true of animals: birds have lower metabolic rates than mammals of the same size. That means birds can run on less fuel for the same mass of living stuff, so birds are a bit more efficient.

So which would you rather be? An efficient engine that does a lot on a little bit of fuel, or a less efficient one that does the same amount of work but takes a lot more fuel?

If you'd rather be the efficient machine, then you'd prefer a lower metabolic rate. If one machine has a higher metabolic rate than another—meaning it uses more fuel, but doesn't get more work done—then the machine with the higher metabolic rate is less efficient than the other and is just wasting fuel.

Since we have to pay for food (fuel) or work to grow it, what good is burning more groceries if we get nothing more out of it? None!

Burning more fuel would be good for someone who is trying to lose weight, since fat is stored fuel. Thus, there's abundant interest in increasing the metabolic rate, at least temporarily. Can you boost your metabolic rate? Yes, you can increase your metabolic rate by doing more work or more exercise. The extra activity burns more fuel, so it's increasing your metabolic rate. Unfortunately, your body tends to compensate for this. The appestat in your brain accounts for the additional fuel needed and adds that demand to your appetite. The result of the appestat's meticulous accounting is that when you eat next, your appetite center will make sure that you replace the extra fuel you burned. Eating on a 3MAD schedule provides the appetite center with plenty of opportunities to drive eating to a level that replaces the extra fuel burned while exercising. It's very difficult to eat on a 3MAD schedule and not eat more to compensate for the extra fuel burned during exercise. That's why there are a lot of people who exercise regularly, even vigorously, but are unable to get rid of the fat they want to lose.

MORE ON METABOLISM

What about the claims of vendors and magazines saying one food or another will "boost your metabolism?"

In most cases the metabolic rate boost that's claimed by the vendor refers only to the increase in gut activity it takes to digest the food. They're referring to an increase in gut activity from digestion that occurs with *any* food.

The digestive process is sort of like bringing home groceries, but all the activity takes place inside your body. Imagine you bring several bags of groceries home. It takes some work to bring the groceries into your kitchen and put them away. The work of putting the groceries away increased your metabolic rate a little as you lifted and moved each item, but what happened to the groceries? Were they used as fuel in the process of putting them away, or were they stored for later use? They were stored, and you burned only a couple of baby-cut carrots' worth of fuel with the work you did putting them away. The gut works the same way, with protein and spices having the most heat-generating effect. Your gut does some work to put away the groceries that you eat, and increases your metabolic rate in the process, but the majority of the calories, like the groceries you bring home, get stored, not burned.

Because every food stimulates digestion and provides fuel for your body, any food can carry the claim of boosting or supporting metabolism! Any food will also boost or support your immune system, because your immune system needs fuel to work. Vendors selling products with "boost" and "support" claims are offering nothing more than what ordinary food does.

Your metabolism is the set of chemical reactions going on in your cells that are required for you to be alive. Can you jump-start it? No. If anyone suggests jump-starting your metabolism, that's a strong clue they're trying to sell you something you don't need. Jump-starting your metabolism would mean your metabolism has stopped. If your metabolism has stopped, you are dead. To meet the jump-start product's claim, it must be able to bring the dead back to life. If you find a food or supplement that can do that, please let me know. Even a cardiac defibrillator's shock to the chest doesn't jump-start metabolism—it only resynchronizes the heartbeat. For the jolt of the shock to do any good, the heart muscle cells must still be alive and have ongoing metabolism.

CONCLUSION

If you see a product claiming to boost, support or jump-start metabolism, translate that to "ignore this advertisement."

Your metabolic rate is the amount of energy your body is using and must be matched by fuel (food) flow to replace the energy it uses. Too much fuel flow for your metabolic rate means the extra fuel gets stored and you gain fat. Too little, and your body uses its fuel reserves (fat) and you lose fat. If your fuel flow and your metabolic rate are in balance, you stay the same. A low metabolic rate isn't a problem if you have the energy and strength you need—it just means your body's more efficient at using fuel.

Activity such as exercise or physically active work increases your total metabolic rate and is essential for good health.

Types of Hunger

Hunger is one of the major obstacles to fat loss, so it's important to recognize that hunger can mean different things. Five different types of hunger can drive overeating.

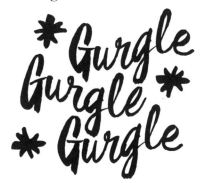

SOMATIC HUNGER

Somatic hunger is the hunger that you feel in your belly; it may feel like sort of a cramping or twisting sensation, and it's often associated with stomach gurgles.

LIMBIC HUNGER

Limbic hunger is the instinctive hunger that drives you to eat more than you intend to eat, as soon as you take the first bite. Limbic hunger is the reason that the serving size on certain thin, minty cookies should be one sleeve, not the four-cookie serving claimed on the package. Limbic hunger is the reason any size bag of chips might become one serving and the potato chip tagline, "nobody can eat just one" generally holds true.

In the survival setting faced by humans for most of the past 100,000 years, limbic hunger made sure that as soon as there was a successful hunt or foraging trip, humans ate more than they needed so that there would be plenty of reserve even if the next meal did not come for several days. Food that wasn't eaten would either rot or be eaten by insects and other animals, so limbic hunger made sure the surplus food/fuel was safely stored in the fat-fridge by prompting more eating than was essential for survival.

CLOCK HUNGER

Clock hunger is your body's biologic clock ticking, saying "Hey, you ate at this time yesterday! Where's today's chow?" Clock hunger is felt as somatic hunger (the feeling in your belly that comes with stomach growls) about 23 – 24 hours after the time you ate the day before. If you eat a morning breakfast, that punches your body clock at that time. The next day at the same time, you'll likely feel hungry, because clock hunger triggers somatic hunger. On the other hand, if you usually eat a morning breakfast, and then don't eat it for several days, your morning breakfast clock hunger will fade, and within a few days, you won't be hungry at that time.

APPETITE-DRIVEN EATING (ADE)

Appetite-driven eating is an odd kind of hunger. You don't feel it as you do somatic hunger, but you can see it and experience it. When you see yourself eating when you'd rather not, that's ADE. You may not even feel any somatic hunger at the time, yet there you are, stuffing food into your mouth when you know you don't need it. Your mind is saying stop, but your body doesn't comply. You'd rather stop eating whatever it is you're eating, but you don't.

MOUTH HUNGER

Mouth hunger is related to ADE. It's the urge to chew on or eat something when you're not really hungry. Mouth hunger may be prompted by eating carbohydrate-rich foods and is distinguished by wanting or craving a particular sensation in the mouth. You don't want to eat just anything; you want something of a particular taste, texture or mouthfeel, such as sweet, crunchy, salty or chewy.

SUMMARY

Hunger isn't just one driving force. There are different kinds and sources, and recognizing them can help you tune into what's prompting you to eat.

Now that you know the terms you need to know for a good understanding of appetite correction, let's take a moment to get rid of some unwanted dead weight of another kind: myths.

Myths

MYTH: BREAKFAST IS THE MOST IMPORTANT MEAL OF THE DAY

The phrase "breakfast is the most important meal of the day" is so frequently used that it's accepted without question—it's pure marketing genius. It's been used to sell billions of dollars' worth of breakfast foods and it encourages many people to eat when they're not even hungry. It's a powerful culture driver born from advertising, not science. The expression has become so deeply entrenched in our everyday language that it's assumed to be common knowledge, and those who question it or deviate from its guidance are considered radical heretics of health. The well-known and often-heeded phrase has no more scientific backing than "Disneyland is the happiest place on Earth" or "Energizer batteries keep going and going."

Breakfast has never been shown to be important or otherwise essential to health unless it's the only meal of the day providing good quality nutrition in adequate quantity.

As long as your diet includes good nutrition and adequate quantity sometime during the day, you can choose when to eat without incurring the wrath of mythical health-stealing breakfast fairies.

MYTH: HYPOGLYCEMIA

Hypoglycemia is the medical term for low blood sugar. Many people have a feeling of weakness and low energy several hours after eating and blame it on hypoglycemia, but this sensation, which is quite real, is almost never caused by low blood sugar. Hypoglycemia has been wrongly blamed for this feeling so often that the sensation in the absence of true hypoglycemia is called "non-hypoglycemia." Non-hypoglycemia is medical jargon meaning "well, it's not true hypoglycemia, but it's a real sensation and we don't know exactly what causes it, so instead of calling it by a term we know to be incorrect (hypoglycemia), we'll label it "something-but-it's-not-hypoglycemia." We don't have a better term for it, so maybe we should invent one. How about calling it the "I've taught my body to fuel up every few hours so I get jitters without a food fix blues?"

Seriously, what would you do if you were in the wild for a day or two? Die after a few hours? No, your body would find its reserve and its ancient survival strength and then power through the challenge.

You can see for yourself by using a glucometer (the blood glucose tester that diabetics use) when the feeling occurs. If you test your blood sugar when you're feeling what you call hypoglycemia, and your blood glucose measures greater than 75 mg/dl (4.2 mmol/L), what you're feeling is non-hypoglycemia. That doesn't mean the feeling isn't real—it's just caused by something other than low glucose. Having the feeling doesn't mean it's impossible to adapt to longer intervals between eating. In fact, you can reliably overcome the feeling by insisting that your body adapt to longer intervals between eating instead of having a constant trickle of food in your gut. If your hypoglycemia is real, see your doctor— true hypoglycemia is rare and may mean that something's wrong that could lead to big problems.

> Non-hypoglycemia is a wimpy weakness you can beat. Your body's better than that.

MYTH: FASTING BURNS MUSCLE

Fasting does not burn muscle unless the fast has been going on for at least two days AND there's no more glycogen stored in the liver AND the blood can't spare any protein. In that case, the tiny bit of glucose that the brain needs can be synthesized from muscle proteins. It's a survival tool, and if survival isn't in question (it's not if you're eating your fill every day), then it doesn't happen. All the other fuel needs of the body can come from fat. This myth came from misreporting and/or misinterpretation of a study of U.S. Army Rangers who had muscle loss when eating once a day for a couple of weeks. Here's the catch: The Rangers were already lean, so they didn't have a lot of fat to burn, and the one meal they were allowed each day provided only about 2,500 calories of energy. The Rangers' hiking, training and exposure to the weather demanded an energy output of up to 10,000 calories per day, so the Rangers endured an energy deficit of about 7,500 calories per day—enough to burn about two pounds of fat every day if they had that much to spare. If they didn't have fat to burn, their energy-starved bodies had nowhere to go for the fuel needed to survive except to nibble away at some muscle. The Rangers were so hungry from working at the extreme energy deficit that some caught and ate wild critters and some went outside the authorized area to sneak in food from nearby stores or neighboring farms.

If you are inactive, your muscles will wither from lack of use.

If your body is burning 10,000 calories per day and you have unrestricted access to food at least once per day, your appetite will make sure you eat 10,000 calories per day, which the Rangers desperately wanted to do but could not.

Although brief periods of fasting won't burn muscle when you're eating your fill every day, the "use it or lose it" principle still applies no matter how often or how much you eat. If you are inactive, your muscles will wither from lack of use whether you're eating 1,000 calories a day or 10,000. Though exercise is not as effective as appetite correction for fat loss, exercise remains a fundamental requirement to achieve or maintain good health.

kle my belt usi... want to play flag football. I wan... ...ravel. I want to run a 5k. I want to be able to wear the... want to feel proud of my body. I want to wear fun clothes... I want to be back in my skinny jeans. I want to run a ma... ...edding tux. I want to buckle my belt using a notch I have... ...ant to waterski on vacation. I want to play flag football. I ...airplane seat so I can travel. I want to run a 5k. I want ...at my favorite store. I want to feel proud of my body. I w... ...ant to swim with my kids. I want to be back in my skinny ... ...ion. I want to wear my wedding tux. I want to buckle my ... ...t used since college. I want to waterski on vacation. I wan... ...ant to fit comfortably in an airplane seat so I can travel. ... ...able to wear the clothes at my favorite store. I want to ... ...ear fun clothes. I want to swim with my kids. I wa... ...I want to wear my wedding ... ...t to waters...

I. LEARNING

Your Goal Body

Why have a goal body instead of a goal weight? Weight isn't a great goal for a couple of reasons. The first reason is that we don't really care what we weigh; we care about how we look, how we feel and the health risks that come from having surplus fat. If we happened to be twice the weight but kept the same size, looked the same and had no increased health risk, would anybody care about weight? If looks, activity and health were not affected by increasing weight, accumulating mass would probably become a sport with a hall of fame honoring the champions of density. If excess weight weren't associated with encumbrance, illness and suboptimal appearance, you might only notice the excess weight when your car was riding low or a vacant elevator's capacity alarm sounded as you stepped aboard. Weight alone would not be a concern—at least not until furniture began breaking under you.

The second reason that weight is not a great goal is that a lot of things influence your weight besides the amount of fat in your body. Your body is 70 percent water. Water enters your body easily as you eat and drink; it makes up a lot of many of the foods you eat. Water is lost through your breath and leaves your body quickly when you're urinating, sweating or having diarrhea. Water is also lost in regular ol' poop. The amount of salt and carbohydrates in your diet can change how much water your body holds, and the fluctuations caused by changes in the water content of your body can shift your weight up and down by more than a pound (0.45 kg) every day. The water eventually balances out—you don't shrivel like a raisin and you don't blow up like a water balloon. Meanwhile, even if you eat nothing for a day, you'll burn less than a pound of fat. If you lose fat at a steady pound-per-week rate, that's only 0.14 pounds (65 g) of fat per day, a change too small to see on most bathroom scales.

Because your body water can shift around more quickly and in greater amounts than fat, a weight change due to water fluctuations can easily hide weight change due to fat loss. That means you can have weight gain even though you've had a fat loss.

> # Because of shifts in water weight, you can have a weight gain even when you've had a fat loss.

Gaining weight while losing fat is discouraging and it may confuse you by suggesting that what you're doing to burn fat is not working when it really is. Tracking fat loss by recording weight is a bit like listening for bird calls at an outdoor rock concert—the birds may be there and their sounds may be there, but there are so many other sources of sound, most of them louder, that birdsongs will be very difficult to detect.

Let's forget about the number on the scale and set your sights on all the really good stuff that comes with achieving your goal body. What is it about being lean that you want? That happy place is sometimes hard to describe, but it can mean you're back in your skinny jeans, or that you can wear the suit/tux you wore for your wedding, or that you buckle your belt using a notch you haven't used since college. Your goal body may be related to an activity you want to do. Is your goal body playing flag football? Compelling a lover's touch? Running a 5K? A marathon? Take a moment to imagine yourself in your goal body.

Write or sketch whatever describes where you'd like to be. _I_magine yourself living your life in your goal body.

There are two other bodies to consider in addition to your goal body. The first is your "not-at-goal" body, meaning the body you have before reaching your goal. There's also the ideal body, which is the best body you can imagine for yourself. Your ideal body may be leaner or more muscular than your goal body, or it may look the same but be in better condition or have new skills in sports, dancing or some other activity. Your ideal body may be the same as your goal body, but it may also be a few stepping stones beyond it. For the sake of brevity (and so it's easier to use as an adjective), I'll abbreviate not-at-goal body as n-body, goal body as g-body and ideal body as i-body.

TO REVIEW, WE HAVE THREE BODIES TO KEEP IN MIND:

- Where you are now: n–body (not at goal—more fat than you want to have)

- Your goal body (g-body), where you'd feel happy with your body.

- Your ideal body (i-body)—the best you can imagine for your body.

   Your g-body may be best reflected in a clothing size, waist circumference, a feeling of lightness on your feet, a particular contour in the image reflected in your mirror or some other measurement. Your g-body may be defined as fitting into a pair of old trousers or a favorite cocktail dress. You can also have stepping stones on your way to your g-body called non-scale victories (NSVs). Some NSVs mentioned by Fast-5ers include:

- Shopping at Men's Wearhouse instead of the Big & Tall store

- Shopping in the misses' section instead of women's or plus sizes

- Fitting into the booths at McDonald's

- Losing the social baggage of being fat

- Increasing your activity because you feel good and strong

- Giving away clothes that are too big, knowing you'll never need them again

- Downsizing your wedding ring because it slips off too easily

- Fitting into a smaller clothing size

- Reaching a pre-pregnancy size

- Tightening your belt a notch

- Hearing a co-worker ask if you've lost weight

- Hearing a co-worker ask how you've lost weight

- Feeling the willpower to pass up a donut at work or popcorn during a movie

- Reaching your college weight

- Having your pants or skirt feel loose or fall down

- Having more cash in your wallet or pocketbook at the end of the week because you no longer buy snacks throughout the day

- Seeing muscles or other body contours that have been hidden for years.

The look, the feel, the responses and the freedom from excess fat are all facets of your g-body.

What does your g-body look like? How does it feel? How do others respond to seeing you in your g-body? What will you do in your g-body that you don't feel like doing right now?

Here are some more reasons why judging fat loss only by weight doesn't work well:

1. If someone starts exercising while losing fat, his or her weight may not drop very much. With muscle mass increasing as fat mass is decreasing, there may not be much progress evident when it's measured by weight. Muscle mass usually won't grow as fast or as much as fat mass can decrease, but the opposing change can hide real progress if you're only paying attention to the scale and not to other changes.

2. Mindset is very important for sustaining any plan. Keeping a g-body in mind means you visualize your g-body along with its associated activities, benefits and freedoms. Your g-body reminds you of how you want to look and feel, and lets you stop chasing a number on the scale. Keeping your real goal in mind instead of a number reflecting a specific weight may help you maintain the endurance necessary to reach your goal. Once you achieve your first goal body, you may find yourself establishing a new goal body—one you previously thought impossible.

3. Sumo wrestlers may be the only people on the planet who choose to be overweight. You didn't. Having numbers on a scale remind you daily that you fall into one class or another of overweight can be frustrating and depressing. Instead of being overweight, you are in your n-body stage—your not-at-goal body. The goal body perspective embodies three important facts: (a) you see your current state (n-body) as a temporary condition; (b) you are not where you want to be, and (c) you are motivated and working to get to your g-body.

4. There are formal definitions for overweight and obesity that make talking about having excess fat awkward or technically incorrect. You are a valid judge of when your body's at its best, so your goal body is the only goal you need.

5. Lots of charts and calculators will tell you an ideal weight, but in real life, it can be very difficult to maintain a lower weight than your body and appetite center will agree to. Your g-body is one that's both satisfying to you and relatively easy to maintain because you're working with your body, not against it.

Focusing on your goal body (g-body) means you can leave the term OVERWEIGHT behind.

I. LEARNING

Weighing In

IF YOU MUST TRACK YOUR WEIGHT

If you feel compelled to establish a goal weight in addition to your goal body, then it makes sense to approach the weighing-in process with understanding and realistic expectations. Keep in mind that progress will look like a very bumpy path with a slight overall downward angle.

When measuring fat loss, ideally we would measure fat, not weight, but there's no easy way to measure just fat. Tape measures work, but they can be awkward, and it may be difficult to measure in exactly the same place each time unless you trace your circumference with a Sharpie. It can also be difficult to know when you've got your belly sucked in as much as you did the last time you measured. If we use weight instead, there's the problem mentioned previously: your weight includes a lot of things besides fat. It includes several gallons of water plus bones and muscle along with what you ate yesterday and maybe the day before.

Even though many scales imply super precision by displaying a digit after the decimal place (such as saying 150.1 pounds or 68.2 kg) they're not a precise measurement of your body fat loss or gain because so much changes in your water-rich body besides fat. A few hours from now—after you use the bathroom or drink a beer or have a meal, your weight may be different on the scale even though your body fat hasn't changed a bit. When it comes to measuring your fat content, ignore the fluctuations in that extra digit; they're to be expected.

Precision is important in a scale, and a scale can have good precision even if it has no digits after the decimal place. You want a scale that's going to say the same thing every time you put an identical weight on it. If you step on a scale, read it, then step off and back on for another reading, a precise scale will read the same weight or vary at most by 0.1 with the repeat measurements. Scales offering body fat measurements provide no real added value because electronic body fat measurement techniques yield highly variable results. As the water shifts mentioned earlier occur, it makes the body fat percentage appear higher (when water is lost) or lower (when water retention is up) when it hasn't actually changed. The devices are more of a gimmick than a tool.

Once you've confirmed that your scale has adequate precision, it's time to weigh, but that may not be as straightforward as you might guess.

Weighing yourself is simple, right? Step on the scale, read, step off. What can go wrong? More than you might think. Here are some suggestions for getting reliable numbers without needlessly frustrating yourself, going bonkers or wasting your time chasing meaningless numbers. Misinterpreting your weight change could lead you to make a wrong decision about whether your effort to lose or maintain weight is working, so it's important to get it right.

Use the same scale for all your measurements. Comparing weights from two scales, even if one is at a doctor's office, is asking for confusion.

For consistency, weigh yourself at the same time of day, preferably in the morning after urinating. Since the water content of your body can cause your weight to fluctuate, weighing after you've been sleeping and after you've emptied your bladder gives your body a chance to get rid of at least some of the excess.

Be realistic about how much fat you can burn in a day. A pound of fat on your body can provide about 2,500–3,500 calories' worth of fuel for your body's functions and activity. That's the same amount of fuel as eating four sticks of butter. Most people burn 1,500–2,500 calories per day and replace that with what they eat. If you don't eat quite enough to replace the loss, say 500 fewer calories than you burn, then your net loss of fat is only 0.14 pounds (0.065 kg) that day. Because the body's fat change is small compared to its water content fluctuations, consistently measuring body weight over the course of several weeks is the only reasonable way to meaningfully track weight. Trends over the course of weeks and months reveal what's really going on in your body. Women may see period-related fluctuations as well, so comparing today's weight to one recorded a week or month ago is more reliable than comparing today's weight to yesterday's.

There are apps and devices available that let you record your weight daily and average it out over several days (called a moving average) so that the fluctuations due to water content are smoothed out. Libra and MyFitnessPal are popular app choices; John Walker's free (and advertisement-free) hackersdiet.com is one of the earliest web-based support apps to emphasize the variable nature of water shifts, and his site includes the moving average feature in online weight loss tracking. A simple alternative to using apps is recording weights daily on a calendar and comparing one day's weight to the same day of the week one week or one month earlier.

EXPECTING TO SEE WEIGHT LOSS FOLLOWING YOUR SWEATY HOUR ON THE TREADMILL?

Don't. Even if you run fast and manage to cover 15 km (9.4 miles) in the hour, your workout will only burn about a third of a pound of fat. Your sweat loss will probably amount to more than that, maybe as much as a pound, but sweating also makes you thirsty. It wouldn't be unusual to drink a liter of water to replace fluid you lost during a vigorous workout. If you do that, you'll add back 2.2 pounds (1 kg) of water to your body and weigh more at the end of your workout than you did when you started.

If you eat following the exercise and before weighing, then your body has the opportunity to replace the used fuel, so even a marathoner may see no measurable weight loss the morning after the big run. Contrary to popular hope, exercise doesn't burn off calories very quickly, and unless you have many hours every day to exercise, cutting calories by eating less is a lot easier than trying to burn off extra calories with exercise. Exercising with the intent to burn off fat can turn into an exercise in frustration because, as mentioned before, the appestat will notch up appetite-driven eating to compensate for energy spent on activities. In the end, you wind up eating a bit more food to replace the fuel you burned off with exercise.

Remember your goal body. Don't let your scale be your only measuring tool.

Notice the fit of your clothes and which notch on your belt you're using. Write it down here or in a notebook so you don't have to wonder later. Feeling a loosening of your clothing can indicate fat loss just as well, if not better, than a scale. If your shorts fall off, you're doing well! If your waistband or belt is getting tighter over the course of 2–3 weeks, it's probably time to change what you're doing.

WEEK	OBSERVATIONS
1	
2	
3	
4	
5	
6	
7	
8	
9	
10	

I. LEARNING

Leverage on the Autopilot

Even though the autopilot systems in the brain core can override your conscious will, it's kind of a two way street. If you want to breathe faster, you can do so. You can increase your breathing rate for a little while just by thinking about it. You can keep your breathing rate up a lot longer if you choose to do something that demands it, like going for a jog. What if you wanted to raise your heart rate? You can't get your heart ticking faster just by willing it, but you can make it happen by exercising or thinking about some exciting event. Within seconds of starting exercise, you can double your heart rate. By initiating a voluntary action, you've changed something that your will alone could not do. Want your heart to beat even faster? Exercise harder. Up it goes. Want it to slow down? All you have to do is back off the exercise.

You can't make it go too fast, and you can't make it go too slowly, but you can change your heart rate through conscious choices. Finding ways to indirectly change things you can't directly control means you're using leverage. Leverage is another way of saying you're using a tool to get the desired effect.

You have leverage on some other automatic body functions. Want to make your pupils dilate? You can't just make them dilate, but you can choose to go into a dark room. Poof! You made your pupils dilate. Want to make them constrict to pinholes? Look at a bright light. Can you make yourself sneeze? Probably not just by thinking about it, but sniffing some pepper might make it happen. If you provoke a sneeze, then your conscious choice has influenced your automatic systems.

Appetite-driven eating is no different. You can't directly adjust your appestat, but by exerting your conscious control on some things, you can influence your appestat so that the amount it drives you to eat is corrected to where it should be. In other words, you can use tools as leverage to help your appestat work like it's supposed to—no more confusion, no more out-of-tune overeating.

Appetite correction (AC) means you lose fat without counting calories or using brute-force willpower.

When you have achieved AC, you eat all you want, but you want less and feel full with less. A corrected appetite may also steer you toward better food choices.

The idea that your appetite can be corrected may sound foreign to you, or even unbelievable, but AC can and does work. When you've achieved AC, there's no longer a need to count calories or summon up willpower. Your appestat does the calorie counting for you. With AC, your appestat works for you in the same way appestats work for all the non-human and non-human-fed animals you see around you. When it's working, you don't eat too much. With AC, if you have surplus fat, you eat a bit less than your body's fuel demand requires until the surplus fat (fuel) has been used up. Once your surplus fat is gone, your appestat automatically increases your appetite a notch, just enough to maintain a steady balance. When it works like it should, the appestat is an amazing system.

Ready to clear out the gremlins that are messing with your appestat? Let's take another quick look at them.

I. LEARNING

Appetite Gremlins

Even though our bodies are our primary vehicles for life, we're not interested in a race to the finish line. No one in good health is particularly eager to end the ride. For our body-vehicles, the important thing is not speeding through life, but enjoying the ride and making sure our individual vehicle provides a fun, reliable ride for as long as possible. We've talked about the many ways that our everyday environment differs from that of non-human animals, and the factors that may promote eating and confuse your appetite. We don't know exactly what all of the causes of confusion are, so we're chalking it up to gremlins tinkering with your vehicle. It's time to talk about how to fix the problem. We're not going to waste time on solutions that cannot be part of your permanent, lifetime solution, and we're not talking about austere measures: no eating bugs and no giving up electricity. If you find it hard to imagine never worrying about calories or fat again, that's understandable, but that's the goal: a naturally lean lifestyle that you can comfortably sustain for the rest of your life.

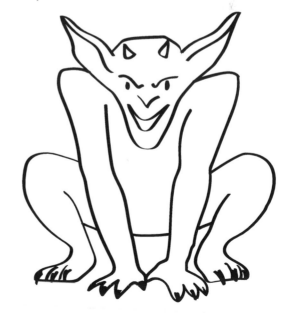

TO REVIEW SOME OF THE COMMON FACTORS THAT MAY BE AMONG THE GREMLINS CONFUSING YOUR APPESTAT, HERE'S A BRIEF LIST:

· Advertising encourages you to eat rich foods and to eat frequently.

· Social occasions are almost always food-centered.

· Meal schedules encourage you to eat regardless of hunger/appetite.

· Food is engineered to be appetite-stimulating.

· Easy access and acquisition of food: You don't have to hunt it, catch it, grow it or gather it. You have your grocery store, pantry, refrigerator and countless other food sources.

· Easy and quick preparation of food thanks to tools: Think about how long it would take to prepare and eat a meal with no knives, pots, blenders, slicers, food processors, mixers, ranges or ovens.

· Ultra-convenient forms of food: Frozen dinners and hundreds of ready-to-eat or nearly-ready-to-eat choices are available in boxes, bags or other packages.

· Fuel bombs: The high calorie concentration in sweets, honey and nuts is no longer offset by a challenge in acquiring them—one does not have to deal with sugar cane, bees or shells.

· High-sugar fruits: Varieties of almost all fruits, including apples and bananas, have been carefully selected and bred since the 1500s. In the last hundred years, advanced techniques have been applied to produce fruit with ever-higher sugar content and longer shelf life to increase the fruit's appeal to shoppers.

· Social pressure: There is high pressure in schools and workplaces to snack.

· Pre-digested foods: Grinding, processing and refining techniques allow for quick eating and complete food absorption.

· Extended day/night cycles: Plentiful, convenient electric lighting disrupts the natural rhythm of our internal clocks.

· Inadequate sleep due to late-night entertainment and awakening to alarm clocks in the morning.

Whatever the actual gremlins are in your case, they have messed with your appestat to the point it's confused. When it's confused, it causes you to gain fat you don't need.

To get your appestat working correctly again, you could push away the gremlins with sheer will, but that's tough. It gets tiring, and even on the best days, gremlins can still sneak in and mess with your appestat. You wouldn't be reading this book if it were an easy fix.

What do we humans do when we know something can be done, but it's hard? We make and use tools! The next section in this book is the AC tool shed, which is like a pit stop for your body-vehicle. The AC tool shed is a selection of non-drug, non-surgical tools available to help push the appestat gremlins away so you can keep your

MY APPETITE GREMLINS

body-vehicle's appestat tuned correctly. The tools you select from the AC tool shed constitute your AC toolkit. You don't have to use all the tools in the shed—sometimes, one good tool is all you need to keep your body-vehicle tuned up.

The tools listed are called tools for a good reason—tools make a tough job easier, but they do nothing by themselves. You have to apply at least a little effort to get something done. It's important that you're comfortable with your AC toolkit, because this is a lifestyle change. AC is not a quick fix, nor is it something you do for a few months and quit. The AC toolkit that makes the best match for your life may take some experimenting to find. Tweaking lets you customize your AC toolkit to create a comfortable fit with your life that you can maintain indefinitely. The tools you choose to use may change over time as your life and needs change.

You may use several tools together to achieve fat loss, then put a few back in the shed when you've reached your goal body and only need to maintain. If your appestat starts acting confused again, the same tools you used before will be there for you when you need them.

How do you know when your AC toolkit is working? You know it's working when you see fat loss, measured as either looser-fitting clothing or lower numbers on the scale, when you haven't really been watching what you eat. That doesn't mean you can eat with wild abandon—it just means you don't have to struggle. Don't expect to see results in a day or two—it takes a minimum of three weeks to get into your AC groove. Your appestat's gremlins didn't all jump on your appestat in one day—they've been sneaking around for years. Don't be surprised if it takes some time to clear them out. You didn't build your fat surplus in a day either, so don't expect it to melt away miraculously—that's another good reason to allow at least a week between measurements. Ready to see what's in the AC tool shed? We're almost there—just one more thing to cover:

Based on experience, I know this next sentence bears repeating, so I'm highlighting it before we even get to the tool shed. **Don't expect AC to work in a day or even three or four! It will take at least three weeks of a lifestyle change to see an effect on your appetite. Trust your body a lot, trust me a little, and you may be surprised at how well your body can work.**

II. DOING

Tool 1: Your Compass

STUDY OF ONE

The first tool in the shed is like a compass or GPS. It allows you to know if you're headed in the right direction. "Study of One" means that you're experimenting on one person—you—and you're looking to see whether a change you've made is doing good stuff for you or not.

There are some unhealthy ways to lose fat, such as drugs, anorexia or bulemia. AC is nothing so extreme, but you still want to be sure it's a healthy choice for you. How can you be sure an AC lifestyle is a healthy choice? Put it to the test! The easiest way to test it is to take a snapshot of your health now so you can compare to it later.

This basic snapshot includes some measurements you take yourself. For extra confidence, you can ask your doctor to help you with some lab tests. This is the first step of a study of one: getting a fix on where you are now so you can tell whether the change you're making is good for you or not.

1. Check your waist measurement by measuring the distance around your belly at your navel. Measure while standing in front of a mirror so you can keep the measuring tape precisely horizontal (parallel to the bottom of the mirror/floor) so you know where to measure next time. Don't hold your belly in at all. That's right, just relax and let it go for this measurement!

2. If you have a scale that passes the precision test described in the "Weighing In" chapter, check your weight and record it, along with how you were dressed when you weighed (clothed, nude, shoes on/off, etc.)

3. Check your blood pressure three times on a drugstore machine or on a home unit. Record all three measurements. If the difference between the systolic (top) numbers varies by more than five between different measurements, take more measurements until you get three values that vary by five or less. When you have your three measurements, determine the average. To do that, add all three systolic (top) numbers together and then divide the total by three. Repeat the process with the diastolic (bottom) numbers. Record the result as your average blood pressure along with the date you took the measurement. When you take your blood pressure next, perhaps a few months from now, use the same device and the same method so you can compare the two averages.

Here's an example using numbers I recorded during one sitting at a machine at a nearby big box store.

Test 1: 101/70

Test 2: 96/72

Test 3: 96/71

Are all the top numbers within five of each other? Yes, the difference between the highest number and the lowest number is five (101 - 96 = 5).

If the difference had been greater than five, I would run the test again until I had three in a row that had a difference of five or less.

Now for the bottom (diastolic) numbers: Is the difference between the highest and lowest diastolic number five or less? Yes! (72 - 70 = 2). First, I add all the top numbers and divide the total by three:

101 + 96 + 96 = 293.

293 divided by 3 = 97.6, which rounds to an average systolic blood pressure of 98.
I then add all the bottom numbers and divide the total by 3:

70 + 71 + 72 = 213.

213 divided by 3 = 71, so that's my average diastolic blood pressure.
Putting the two numbers together, my average blood pressure (BP) is 98/71 for this measurement.

4. If you want before-and-after pictures, now's the time to take the "before" photo. Whether it's a selfie, self-timed, or someone takes it for you doesn't matter, but make sure your setup is something you can duplicate later. Take your picture wearing the least amount of clothing

you find comfortable. Wear clothing that is snug, but avoid very tight clothing or spandex shapewear so you get an authentic look. Note your position and the position of the camera so you can reproduce the same angles and perspective in later comparison shots.

5. With a doctor's help, you can check some other general health indicators: your HS-CRP, HbA1c and lipid profile.

HS-CRP is a measure of the overall level of inflammation in your body. If you have some obvious source of inflammation, for example, if you're fighting a cold or you've twisted your ankle and it's still swollen, wait until that subsides before checking your HS-CRP. The lower your HS-CRP is, the better.

HbA1c is a measure of the average blood glucose level over the course of a couple of months. As with HS-CRP, the lower the HbA1c, the better.

The lipid profile is an indicator of your risk for heart and blood vessel disease. Two numbers in the lipid profile that are good to follow include the total cholesterol and the cholesterol/HDL ratio (lower is better).

Your doctor will likely have some other guidance to add, and may be able to offer a perspective on how you're doing compared to others in your community who eat similar foods in a similar environment.

You don't have to have these lab tests to start an AC lifestyle, but seeing improvement in these numbers can be great encouragement and can let you know with some concrete evidence whether a change you make in your lifestyle is healthier than what you were doing previously. It's also great to have your own numbers and results so you can scuttle criticism and fend off the flak that others might bring forward. When people start to notice that you're losing weight and that you're not struggling or depriving yourself in the process, you may encounter a naysayer or two offering authoritative advice about what you should or shouldn't be doing.

Many a seasoned and successful Fast-5er has endured a host of criticisms based on advertising-driven notions like "everyone knows" and marketing gems like "breakfast is the most important meal of the day."

People can be quick to share information from studies they've heard about but have never looked at. When that happens, it's helpful to remind yourself that you're testing AC with your own study of one. If your inflammation is down, your blood glucose is down (the opposite of diabetes) and your doctor's giving you the thumbs-up on your cholesterol levels, let your critics grumble while you're losing fat and feeling great about yourself and your future.

When you're evaluating the health of your current AC lifestyle, don't compare the test results to some healthy ideal or "normal" range that you may have never achieved. Instead, compare it to your previous results so that you are comparing your present condition to your past condition. That's why it's important to get a navigational fix on your health before you start an AC lifestyle.

For example, if your current waist circumference is 40 inches (102 cm), don't compare that to your ideal of maybe 24 inches (61 cm) or 30 inches (76 cm) and say "well, that's not healthy!" Compare it instead to where you've been. If you were at 42 inches (107 cm) before starting your AC lifestyle, then you're seeing a healthy change. The same goes for lab tests. If you see your HS-CRP at 3.0 mg/L, you have to know where it was before to know whether you're heading in the right direction. A lower HS-CRP is better, so if it was at 6.0 mg/L previously, your choices are looking good, but if it was at 1.0 mg/L, it may be time to re-examine your choices.

TOOL SUMMARY:

Like a compass or GPS, recording some information now starts your Study of One. The information gives you a waypoint—something to compare to later, so you can wisely navigate your AC lifestyle. In a few months, you'll compare new information to this reference point to determine whether your AC lifestyle is healthier than what you were doing before.

II. DOING

Tool 2: ACES

APPETITE CORRECTING EATING SCHEDULE

If we don't know what's confusing the appetite center, is the solution to go primitive and eat like animals—raw food with no schedule? That might work if we lived in a culture in which you could eat exclusively according to your need and ignore the 3MAD schedule along with other social cues that either prompt or demand eating. Unfortunately for humans with surplus fat, eating on a schedule is a deeply ingrained custom in our culture. Many social practices center on eating. Birthdays wouldn't be birthdays without cake! Our celebratory instincts involve food and/or drink as they have for thousands of years.

Fortunately, there is a way to get the appetite center working as it should without becoming a raw-food animal isolated from human cultural customs and social opportunities. Ironically, the solution to appestat confusion caused by eating on a schedule is to eat on a different schedule.

COMPONENTS

The AC eating schedule starts with the same schedule rule that Fast-5 has (eat within five consecutive hours) and adds a note, a prediction, a test and a term, conveniently bringing the total number of components in this powerful AC tool to a total of five. Here they are:

THE NOTE

Expect no fat loss before or during the adaptation period; you may even gain some. There is an adjustment period of about three weeks that starts the first day you eat only within your selected five-hour window. During this three-week adaptation period, the "magic" that makes an appetite correcting schedule work begins. When eating on an AC schedule, the appestat recognizes how much fat you have stored on your body and guides your food consumption accordingly. As the appestat resets, the quantity of food you desire drops, so your calorie intake falls. When your appestat resets, you eat less—not because you're working to limit calories and saying "no" to yourself, but because you don't want to eat as much as you did before.

During the three-week adaptation period, you gain confidence in your body's ability to go a few extra hours without eating. At the same time, compensatory overeating (eating extra because you think you must to avoid hunger the next day) fades away.

If you lose some fat or water weight during the first weeks, that doesn't mean something is broken—it's a good thing and can be very encouraging. Water weight may come off quickly during the first few days and weeks of an AC eating schedule, but don't expect that rate of loss to continue. It can't continue and it won't, but it is real weight that you want to lose, so it's great to see it go!

THE PREDICTION

The ACES prediction is that your average fat loss will be a pound (0.45 kg) per week starting after the three-week adaptation period and continuing to your goal. Some people see a bit more, others a bit less, and you may see periods of a few weeks without fat loss called plateaus. This AC prediction gives you some idea how long it may take to reach your goal. Fat loss progress may be uneven, so you may lose two pounds one week, then none the next. This prediction is an average of a pound per week over the course of several weeks, not a fixed amount every week.

THE TEST

The ACES Test is the question "Does it work for you?" This test applies to any modifications (tweaks) you might want to make to the AC eating schedule rule. If the change works for you, that's great! If it doesn't work for you, then it doesn't matter if it works for someone else or not. What if your tweak works for you but doesn't work for anyone else in the whole world? That doesn't matter, either—if it works for you, keep it up! By applying this test to any tweaks you make, you can find the AC lifestyle that fits your life the best. Tweaking is best started after steady fat loss is underway so you

---

can be sure the basic AC eating schedule works for you before you start modifying it. It takes two to three weeks for changes to show an effect, so give each tweak you make a three-week trial before applying the AC test: "Does it work for you?"

Fasting means no eating and zero calorie intake. Can you get away with five calories' worth of cream in your coffee? What about ten? Twenty? What about coconut oil? Or a protein supplement? Or celery? Or branched-chain amino acids (BCAAs)? All those things include eating or have calories, so they're tweaks. Apply the AC test (Does it work for you?) and you'll find your personalized answer to all the questions that start with "Can I eat. . .?" and "Can I take. . .?"

THE TERM: ACES

ACES is short for appetite correcting eating schedule. Since 2005 when the Fast-5 book was published, the number one difficulty that people have encountered in adopting a Fast-5 schedule has not been hunger, lack of willpower or lack of energy as you might expect. In fact, most people report an increase in energy and have been surprised at the willpower they find they have when they're outside of the eating window. The number one obstacle to adopting and feeling comfortable on the Fast-5

schedule has been the criticism of others who are unfamiliar with the numerous scientifically verified benefits of fasting.

To avoid the abundant flak that bubbles up from ignorance, use words other than fasting to describe your schedule. Fasting is laden with cultural baggage that evokes images of bony, sickly people who aren't much fun to be around. That sort of image causes uninformed people to cringe and think that frailty, anorexia and a sour mood are inevitable for anyone doing any sort of fasting. The scientific term for eating on a schedule with extended intervals between meals is intermittent fasting (IF). Using the term intermittent fasting, though, may be doubly provocative of criticism among the general public because the word intermittent is widely understood to mean unpredictable and unreliable—not just interrupted. Those who have adopted an IF lifestyle know well that IF is quite the opposite: IF is predictable and reliable.

The flak that you may encounter about fasting is understandable. After all, an unreliable and unpredictable regimen of not eating does sound sort of unhealthy, doesn't it? People whose knowledge of health and nutrition comes from TV ads and a "telephone game" of stale dogma passed along through a long line of people in schools, gyms, clinics and media channels don't recognize what they're swallowing. The nutritional gospel they believe in so strongly has been force-fed to them by corporations who are paying media channels big bucks for the opportunity to blast the audience with a point of view intended to sell something. When the only thing people hear is this PR-promoted propaganda, they have no way of knowing that they're getting a one-sided story, a story designed to persuade them to buy something. They have no way of knowing that loads of inconvenient information that scuttles the claims of advertisers selling such things as supplements, gym memberships or equipment and other weight loss products remains buried in journals.

Many people assume that some reliable authority vets the information presented on television, but that's no more true for television than it is for the Internet. The effect of one-sided, advertising-driven information is magnified by our culture's insistence that eating a lot is a sign of good health, as seen the the phrase "he has a healthy appetite." This "eating a lot means you're healthy" mindset endures despite evidence visible to all that our culture is collapsing under an epidemic of obesity and diabetes from out-of-tune appetites driving people to eat quantities of food that are clearly both excessive and unhealthy.

For example, poorly designed studies suggesting that breakfast is a healthy choice get pushed to the public via the media by cereal company public relations (PR) teams. When a more scientifically valid study showing that breakfast doesn't matter is published, it doesn't get the same hype. No company can leverage skipping breakfast into increased sales. On the other hand, positive spin on the benefits of breakfast can have breakfast selling like...well, hotcakes! There's no PR push behind the contrary information because there's nothing to sell.

Cut the critics a break—they don't know what they don't know. You can waste a lot of time and alienate people trying to educate them or you can simply allow your results to speak for themselves. Over time, your success, your experience and your measurements will be all the proof of health you need.

Another term for short-interval intermittent fasting with fasting periods of less than a day is "time restricted feeding." Although the term avoids some of the emotionally laden reputation of fasting, it unfortunately sounds like you eat whenever the zookeeper gets around to sliding a bowl of chow through the bars of your cage.

You're not in a cage, you're in control. Instead of using rant-provoking terms like fasting, you may prefer to unleash positive ACES terminology. To anyone who asks why you're not eating, answer with the phrase

"I'm on an appetite-correcting eating schedule," or "I'm not in my eating window."

That sends a clear message: yes, you eat. You eat as much as you want to. You ate earlier and you'll eat later, but you don't happen to be eating right now.

Using "appetite correcting eating schedule" to describe your particular variety of eating lifestyle can help keep the flak to a minimum until your results can speak for themselves. Soon, your growing confidence in your body will let you brush off the flak as the misinformation born of ignorance and infoclutter that it is. With appetite correcting eating schedules growing in popularity, it is becoming easier to adopt one because the ignorance about fasting is being replaced with real-world awareness, results and information.

HOW DOES AN AC EATING SCHEDULE CORRECT THE APPESTAT?

The details of how the appestat is recalibrated by a schedule change are not yet clear, but we have a couple of clues. The fasting interval of 19 hours, repeated daily, is adequate to create ketosis. Ketosis refers to the presence of ketones in the blood and is not the same as ketoacidosis, a dangerous condition that occurs in diabetics. Ketones are made by the liver when fat is burned as fuel, so the presence of ketones in the blood, urine or breath indicates that one is in or has recently been in a fat-burning state. When ketones are generated by the liver, they circulate in the blood and can be used as fuel by muscle, brain and other tissues. Ketones can be measured in the blood, urine (using Ketostix strips), or breath (using a Ketonix breath analyzer).

Fat is an organ that communicates with the gut, brain and other fat cells using over 40 different hormones. Fat maintains a continuous conversation with these other tissues to regulate the storage and release of fuel in the form of fat. Some of the hormones have been identified and show some role in appetite control. Ketones, or something produced along with them, may be a part of the conversation that tells the appestat how much fat is available. The fasting period may provide the appestat with a true zero point for calorie absorption, without which it misreads the number of calories absorbed from the gut. The full picture of how ACES helps the appetite center find the proper tuning and correct intake isn't clear.

HEY, 19?

The AC eating schedule of 19 hours of fasting with a five-hour eating window can be abbreviated as 19/5. Why start at 19/5 and not 18/6 or 20/4? It's a good question. After all, we said real fasting starts at about 18 hours. The answer is that through the first ten years of experience with Fast-5, the 19/5 schedule has been the just-right "Goldilocks" zone of what works while remaining compatible with real life for real people in the real world. One of the reasons the schedule has worked as well as it has is that it has built-in slip room. If you aim for the 19-hour fast and hit it most days but slip a little here and there, you still are likely to see its remarkable power of appetite correction. That may not happen at 18/6 or 16/8 and if it works at 19/5, there's no reason to make it more austere at 20/4.

A few people starting Fast-5 experienced AC only after shortening the eating window (to 20/4 or 21/3), and some went all the way to a single daily meal (23/1), but based on the ten-year experience with Fast-5, ninety percent or more will see the AC effect at 19/5.

MORE ABOUT KETONES

The presence of ketones is strong evidence of fat burning, but they can have a downside. Because they can pass from blood through the lungs into the exhaled breath, ketones can produce a scent that strikes different people in different ways. The odor is sometimes described to be fruity; it may smell like fingernail polish remover, because one of the ketones produced is acetone—the primary ingredient in fingernail polish remover. Some people sense a metallic or other unusual taste when in ketosis, and some describe the scent as bad breath.

As your body ramps up its ability to produce ketones, after several days to a few weeks, it will also increase its ability to burn ketones as fuel. Surplus ketones will initially circulate in your bloodstream and spill over into your urine and breath, but as you adapt to the lifestyle, they will instead be immediately gobbled up by your ketone-burning muscle cells and other tissues.

Because of the increased use, ketone levels in the blood drop, so there is less to spill over into the urine and breath, and while they may still be detectable, they're much less noticeable.

ACES 19/5 IS THE STARTING POINT

Your AC eating schedule isn't limited to 19 hours of fasting and a five-hour eating window (19/5). If a daily eighteen-hour fast and six-hour eating window works to correct your appetite, then that can be your AC eating schedule, abbreviated as 18/6. If you find better results with an eating window of four hours instead of five and that's what it takes to keep your appetite center working correctly, your AC eating schedule is 20/4.

Some intermittent fasting programs have encouraged a weekly cycle instead of a daily one. The positive terms of appetite correction (AC) and appetite correcting eating schedule (ACES) can apply to any schedule that works to correct your appetite. Some people have combined Fast-5 with other schedules like 5:2 to create their own AC plan, and by doing so have found something that works and a schedule they can comfortably maintain indefinitely. If you have an interest in learning more about the 5:2 regimen, there is reference information later in this book.

You determine whether your schedule qualifies as AC by this simple test: If your eating schedule works to correct your appetite so you eat an amount appropriate for your body's fat content without having to fight with sheer willpower, it's AC.

If you have excess fat and you're not losing a little each week, then your eating schedule is not AC for you, even if it worked as AC for someone else.

For some people, the appetite center works just fine with three meals a day. A person eating three meals a day and maintaining ideal body fat content can call that AC too, because AC and ACES refer to any schedule that allows a person's appetite center to adjust intake to attain and maintain goal body status.

WHAT'S YOUR WINDOW?

To get started on an AC eating schedule, choose your daily five-hour eating window. The most popular windows are 1 pm – 6 pm (1300 – 1800), 3 pm – 8 pm (1500 – 2000) and 5 pm – 10 pm (1700 – 2200), but some people use a window in the morning. Most people find it best to open their eating window at the same time every day, and to choose a time that includes the most family and social contact time. There are other possibilities like sliding windows and off-schedule days we'll talk about later, but for now, keep it simple:

> **Select the five-hour window that best suits your work, family, social and leisure needs.**

THE LACK OF RULES FOR AN AC EATING SCHEDULE SOMETIMES THROWS PEOPLE OFF, SO HERE ARE SOME NON-RULES:

- You do not have to eat at the beginning of your window—it's an opportunity to eat, not an obligation.
- There is no required minimum calorie intake during your window. If you don't feel like eating at all, it's okay to extend your fast by a day.
- You don't have to start with a five-hour window.

Experience with Fast-5 indicates that a five-hour window works for almost everyone who tries it, so a five-hour window remains the recommended place to start your AC eating schedule. You can customize your window to fit your schedule and, as long as it still works for you, there's no problem. You can try a window of four hours or six or even eight. If you start with a window longer than five hours and don't see steady fat loss after a few weeks, don't give up on an AC eating schedule until you've shortened your window to five hours or less and have given the five-hour window a four-week try (allowing for three weeks of adaptation for appetite correction and one week in which you can expect to see its effect).

GETTING STARTED WITH ACES

After choosing the time for your window, it's time to get started. The start is the second hardest part of an AC eating schedule (flak from others is the hardest, and we'll talk some more about how to deal with that later.) The start is what pushes your body to use fat for fuel instead of depending on a constant trickle of fuel from your gut. Running mostly on fat is something your body can do very well, but it hasn't been asked to do it much.

Your AC eating schedule is a tool, and as with any tool, it does nothing unless you put it to work. With your effort in your starting push, changes happen and the appetite reset that makes the AC eating schedule work starts to kick in. It doesn't usually kick in fully until you've maintained the schedule for about three weeks. Don't worry about how much you're eating until you've passed the three-week mark. It's typical to eat a little (or a lot) extra at first because you think you're going to be hungry the next day. That's compensatory overeating and it's normal; it usually subsides over the three-week adaptation period.

People start an AC eating schedule in a number of ways; the three most common are cold turkey, ratchet and progressive starts. Use any of these methods, combine them or invent your own path.

No matter which way you start, keep this in mind: if you slip and don't reach your goal, don't give up! Getting close to your goal still pushes your body to adapt, which makes it easier to reach your goal on your next try. Slips are a normal part of adjustment. It's like climbing to the top of a sand dune: as you climb, you expect to slip, and you may slip a lot. If you ignore the slips and keep scrambling up the dune, what is the inevitable result? Success!

A word to know: break-fast. The first time you eat, no matter whether it's morning, afternoon or night, breaks your fast, so we call it break-fast. To avoid confusion with the morning meal, "break-fast" is pronounced like "brake-fast."

THE COLD TURKEY START

In a cold turkey start, you choose on day 1 to not eat until your eating window opens. This approach is usually effective, especially for earlier windows, but may require a number of close-but-not-quite days before you finally reach your target time, especially if your target window starts later in the day. When using this approach, the third, fourth or fifth day is typically a crunch day—the hardest to get through due to hunger. After the crunch day, the days get easier quickly. The crunch day is critical to getting your body to rev up its fat-burning capability. It's just like a workout with weights: you have to push your body for it to build up its ability to do more. When it responds, you can do more than you could before, and that's a wonderful feeling.

Cold Turkey Example

With a window of 3 – 8 pm (1500 – 2000) in mind, Kelly skips breakfast and lunch on day 1, then grabs a snack at 3 pm (1500), has a nice dinner at 6:30 (1830) and doesn't eat anything after 8 pm (2000). The same schedule is repeated on day 2 and continues on day 3, and so on from there. By day 6, Kelly is feeling much less hunger and is easily reaching the window opening time.

THE RATCHET START

To use the ratchet start, push your break-fast time on day 1 at least 15 minutes later than the day before. If you're not hungry, you wait until you are hungry before eating. The next day, set break-fast 15 minutes later, but again, wait until you are truly hungry before eating. This way, your break-fast time moves later in the day as far as you can comfortably push it, but it doesn't fall back. With this approach, you postpone break-fast by whatever time increment your body's ready for. On some days break-fast may be 15 minutes later than the day before, and on other days it may be an hour or more later, but it never falls back. The window closes at the same time every day at the chosen closing time.

As with the cold turkey approach, if you slip and don't reach your goal, don't give up; keep trying until you reach your goal.

Ratchet Example

Alex likes to have a glass of wine in the late evening and likes going out to dinner with friends, so she chooses a 5 pm – 10 pm window (1700 – 2200). On day 1, Alex skips her usual breakfast at 7 am, but gets pretty hungry by 10 am and breaks her fast at 10:30 am. Alex eats according to appetite after that, but doesn't eat after 10 pm (2200), the closing time on her selected window. On day 2, Alex's earliest window-opening option is 10:45 because she wants to stretch past when she broke her fast the day before. At 10:45, she isn't really hungry, so she waits. By 11:45, she's feeling pretty hungry and has break-fast at lunchtime. On day 3, her break-fast is ratcheted fifteen minutes later than the day before, so now she'll break her fast at noon at the earliest. Noon comes, but she's busy and doesn't break her fast until 1 pm (1300). She eats according to her appetite for the rest of day 3 until her window closes at 10 pm (2200). On day 4, the earliest she'll allow herself break-fast is 1:15 pm (1315), 15 minutes after she broke her fast on day 3. On day 4, Alex doesn't feel very hungry until 2:30 (1430), so she breaks her fast then, setting her earliest break-fast for day 5 at 2:45 pm (1445). Alex keeps ratcheting her break-fast time later in the day until she's breaking her fast at her preferred window-opening time of 5 pm (1700) or later.

PROGRESSIVE START

Using progressive adaptation, break-fast is gradually pushed later by the same amount of time every day or every few days until it is the desired window opening time.

Progressive Example

Jim selects a window of 3 – 8 pm (1500 – 2000) with a progressive start on Monday. His usual breakfast time is 7 am (0700), so he sets his first increment of 30 minutes, making his break-fast time at 7:30. He eats according to his appetite until 8 pm (2000), the closing time for his planned window. On Tuesday, he breaks his fast at 8:00 am, on Wednesday at 8:30, Thursday at 9:00, Friday at 9:30 and keeps pushing back his break-fast time by a half hour each day until he is breaking his fast at his planned window opening time of 3 pm (1500).

SLIPPING

Slipping is a natural part of adjusting to an AC eating schedule, both in adjustment and in maintaining the lifestyle. As long as you keep a fasting pattern, a slip or an early break-fast for a social occasion won't cause your body to immediately lose its adaptation to fasting—it takes a few days of not fasting for that to happen. If you break your fast early one day, it may cause you to feel clock hunger (described in more detail in the Learning section on page 36) at the same time the next day—23 to 24 hours later. If you ignore the clock hunger or tell your body that break-fast isn't until your usual break-fast time, the hunger will usually pass fairly quickly, especially if you find something to do as a distraction.

EATING WITHIN YOUR WINDOW

What to Eat

It may be hard to believe, but a lifestyle that includes an AC eating schedule doesn't impose rules about what to eat. That means nothing is off-limits; nothing is taboo. Yes, that means you can have chocolate, wine, beer and pizza! You're a grown-up, so you already know the basics of a healthy diet and you can decide for yourself what's healthy. An AC eating schedule can work with all dietary preferences including omnivore, vegetarian, vegan, kosher, halal, low-carb and paleo. This liberty means you can also incorporate specific diets such as Dr. Joel Fuhrman's nutritarian diet, Dr. Arthur Agatston's South Beach diet, Dr. Dean Ornish's guidelines, the late Dr. Atkins' low-carb regimen or any other plan that specifies dietary content. Low-carb diets work very well in conjunction with an AC eating schedule. When you reach your goal, you can integrate more balanced content. The specifics of optimal intake are not "need-to-know" information to get started, so we'll talk more about what to eat later.

When to Eat

The eating window is the opportunity to eat, not an obligation—the idea is not to eat continuously throughout the window. Some people on a daily AC eating schedule eat a large meal early in the window, and then they snack as desired through the remainder. Others have an early snack or light meal, then a later meal, while some choose to graze through the window. How you distribute your eating through your window is entirely up to you. You will find the way that works best for

you, your body, your schedule, your family and your life. You can also apply the Meal Dynamics tool covered later in this book to manage eating within your window. Theoretically, the ideal way to eat during your window is grazing through small portions until your appetite is satisfied. Stretching your intake over the window results in the lowest insulin peaks and causes the smallest amount of stomach stretching so it stays small and provides a strong "full" sensation with a modest meal. The slow pace also gives your body ample time to measure how much you've eaten. However, grazing may be difficult to maintain as a practice due to prevailing meal-oriented customs and time/convenience issues.

TIMING & EXPECTATIONS

Starting and progressing on an AC eating schedule looks like this:

Start-up: The time it takes to get on the schedule. The start-up duration can range from one day with a cold turkey start to as much as a month with a very gradual progressive start.

Adaptation: A three-week period that starts the first day you eat within your AC schedule's window. It is during this period that compensatory overeating fades away and appetite begins to reset. No weight loss is expected during this time.

Active Loss: The duration of the active loss phase depends on how much fat you have to lose. Expect it to take a week for every pound of fat you want to lose. As you approach your goal body, your appestat will automatically increase your food intake so you stop losing fat and maintain a healthy level of fat reserve, just as if your body were on autopilot—because it is.

Maintenance: In this phase, you're maintaining your goal body after you've lost all the fat you want to lose. You can keep the same AC eating schedule or open the window a little wider. If you start gaining fat, you've opened your window too far; go back to what worked for you.

REASONABLE EXPECTATIONS

It's important to understand what to expect from your AC eating schedule. Some people start an AC eating schedule and quit after a few days because they don't see weight loss or maybe they have gained a little. By giving up on their bodies so quickly because of unrealistic expectations, they lose more than they realize: they lose the potential to see a dream come true. Fat loss shouldn't be expected until after the third week of steady adherence to an AC eating schedule. An AC eating schedule is not a crash diet; it's the tortoise in the tortoise-and-hare parable. It works slowly but steadily, and yes, it wins the race. As the AC prediction says, the typical rate of fat loss is one pound per week. That may not sound like much, but 52 pounds per year is achievable and some have lost quite a bit more. Fifty pounds is far more than most people lose on conventional, commercial diet plans.

During your first week or two on an AC eating schedule, you may see rapid weight loss of up to several pounds. This rapid, early loss is water weight. The loss is largely the result of decreased insulin in your blood. Insulin stimulates the kidneys to retain water, so when insulin falls, the kidneys let more water filter out of your blood and release it as urine. Don't expect that rapid weight loss to continue—it can't. If you've been on another intermittent fasting program or on a low-carb regimen before starting your AC eating schedule, you're unlikely to see rapid water weight loss because your insulin levels have already been reduced.

An AC eating schedule can help you lose fat even if you've never been successful before, but it can't drop 50 pounds by Tuesday like some grocery store check-out tabloids claim—unless it's Tuesday 50 weeks from now!

You may see changes in measurements or looser clothing before seeing a drop in weight, so don't worry if your clothes feel looser but your weight hasn't changed. That's typical, and it's a clear indicator that you're mobilizing fat. To fuel your body's energy needs, fat may be redistributed from bulky depots like your hips and belly to muscles throughout your body where it's going to be used as fuel.

BADGER MANAGEMENT

As I mentioned in the introduction, the most common and most difficult obstacle to overcome in adapting to an AC eating schedule is not hunger. Hunger is usually a distant third—fortunately for most people, it's just a minor bump in the road on the way to full adaptation. The real obstacles are (1) the pile of criticism and judgment that many people are ready to dump on you simply because you're choosing to not eat for a few extra hours each day and (2) the awkwardness and discomfort of socializing without eating. Thanks to recent publicity and wider acceptance of intermittent fasting in recent years, the badgering is not as prevalent or harsh as it used to be, but it is still a significant barrier. Many people following an AC eating schedule keep mum about how they're losing weight.

One of the reasons that the badgering is so common is that most of the dietary information in the public realm has been put there with the intent to sell something (food, supplements or whatever), so it's laden with comments like "Eat this fat-burning food!" and "Boost your metabolism!" to prompt a purchase, then consumption and then yet another purchase. Another reason badgering is common in our food-centered land of plenty: people have rarely gone more than a few hours without food. They haven't tried it, so they have no idea how remarkably resilient and strong the average human body is—even theirs! Many people fear that they couldn't handle such a schedule, and that fear provokes thoughts that what you're doing must carry some threat that would make it not worth doing. It may help to reassure the badger that an AC eating schedule doesn't take exceptional willpower or self-denial.

To help dismantle the dogma that puts the badgers on the attack, I offer these points for "frequently heard badgering…"

Attack: Fasting will slow down your metabolism.

Defense: Fasting doesn't slow down metabolism unless it's maintained for at least 48 hours. Besides, there may be a correlation between lower metabolic rates and living longer compared to those with higher rates. I'll eat less, save money on food while doing all the things I want to do and I may live longer because of it, too. Stuff that in your brain if there's room with all the junk information your TV and all the hype-mongers have put in there.

Attack: You can't get all the nutrients you need in that short time without stuffing yourself.

Defense: Ten pounds of fat is enough fuel to supply all the energy my body needs for at least two weeks even if I eat nothing at all! With the energy coming from my fat, I only have to replace protein, and I don't need much of that since I'm neither growing nor pregnant and protein gets recycled. The recycling can help clean up my cells, which may help them run more cleanly. Recycling protein may be one of the reasons that animals fed less live longer than those with unrestricted access to food.

Attack: You'll binge or become anorexic.

Defense: I may have little binges at first when I'm adjusting, but it passes when I learn to trust that my body has the fuel I need. As for anorexia? I'll stop if lack of appetite ever becomes my problem, but right now, I'm dealing with the problem that I actually have. That's like suggesting I shouldn't wash a dirty pan because I might scrub the bottom out of it.

Attack: It's not a healthy way to eat.

Defense: Eating three meals a day made me and two-thirds of the United States population overweight or obese. That's clearly not healthy. Obesity increases the risk of nine of the top ten causes of death. By dropping my excess weight, I'm reducing that risk, so that's a healthy way to eat. Besides, the three-meal-a-day custom was not developed based on scientific studies—it was spawned by marketing, religious practices and mimicry of rich people who were demonstrating their wealth by consuming multiple meals.

Attack: It'll lead to yo-yo dieting. You may lose, but you'll gain it all right back, and then some.

Defense: That's why it's called a lifestyle. It can be maintained indefinitely, so I don't have to go back to what caused weight gain in the first place. No yo-yo.

Attack: You won't have any energy. You have to eat to keep your brain supplied with fuel.

Defense: People don't lose consciousness when they go a few hours without eating. If you sleep eight hours without setting an alarm to wake up and eat, will you die? We're not fragile! Ancient humans had to go for days without food and were still able to hunt and gather. Fat can supply almost all the energy the body needs, and when my body is running on fat as its main fuel, that means more glucose is available for my brain. It also means I have a steady supply of energy all day long with no after-meal sleepiness. I'm sharper, not slower.

Attack: (from a lean person) You shouldn't have to go so long between meals.

Defense: Can you eat all the time and not gain weight? No? So you're eating on a schedule that keeps your appetite and fat where you want it, right? I'm doing the same thing, it's just a different schedule.

Attack: (from a person with surplus fat) [Insert any piece of fat-loss advice or instruction here]

Defense: How is that working for you?

Attack: (from a person with surplus fat): [Insert any negative comment here]

Defense: Why the hostility? Are you afraid I'll get lean and you won't because you're afraid you're too weak-willed to do what's working for me? Cheer up and peace out, because your body's stronger than you realize and going longer between meals is a lot easier than it sounds!

THINGS REPORTED

These symptoms have all been reported by people adopting an AC eating schedule and may be encountered with any effective AC eating schedule. When science catches up with practice and explains the body's amazing power to correct an out of tune appestat with scheduled eating, we may learn that appetite correction is caused by the same factors that lead to the effects and side effects. Humans are complex systems, and it's amazing how many observable things can change with a minor schedule change. Some of these changes may be coincidental (occurring after starting the schedule, but not caused by it) or they may be outcomes caused by the schedule change.

COMMONLY REPORTED:

- Feeling cool or cold during fasting

- Feeling hot after eating

- Happier, more resilient mood

- More energy

- Increased mental clarity

- More interest in healthier food choices

- Less frequent illness, quicker recovery and relatively mild symptoms when ill compared to peers/family members

- Reduced symptoms of inflammation:

  - allergies

  - asthma

  - eczema

  - irritable bowel syndrome

  - multiple sclerosis

  - joint pain

- Changes in sleep: (usually transient and normalizing over 1 – 2 weeks)

- Insomnia (inability to sleep)

- Sleepiness

- Vivid and/or unusual dreams

- Getting up to urinate (during adaptation)

- Decluttering other aspects of life and home

A new interest and drive to declutter? From a modest change in schedule? Seriously? Yes, seriously! Many people who have adopted an AC eating schedule have reported a strong, new interest in decluttering the home and life. This is usually a good thing, but your spouse, partner or roommate may not be ready to throw out or give away as much as you are.

OCCASIONALLY REPORTED:

- Less heartburn or GERD (gastro-esophageal reflux disease)

- More heartburn or GERD

- Less frequent bowel movements (usually in the first 1 – 2 weeks)

- Fewer headaches

- Lighter periods

- Irregular periods during adaptation

- Longer cycle between periods

- Reduced menstrual discomfort and cramping

RARELY REPORTED:

- Less energy

- Less endurance

- More endurance

- Irritability (usually during adaptation)

- More frequent bowel movements and/
  or diarrhea resolving within 1 - 2 days

- Mental fog (usually during adaptation)

- Lightheadedness, especially during adaptation

- More headaches (during adaptation)

GALLSTONES/
GALLBLADDER PROBLEMS

The gallbladder stores bile that's been made by the liver. During digestion, the gallbladder injects the stored bile into the small intestine to help with digestion. Gallstones (also known as calculi) sometimes form in the gallbladder. The gallstones form more frequently in people with excess fat, and rapid weight loss may either enhance formation of gallstones, increase the risk of problems from gallstones, or both. Gallstones may loiter in the gallbladder causing no trouble, but they can also get stuck in the tube that carries the bile from the gallbladder into the small intestine, causing significant pain and possibly other serious problems. The frequency with which gallstones dissolve on their own after excess fat is lost is not known.

FEELING COLDER THAN
YOUR COLLEAGUES

Feeling cool when others are comfortable is a common observation among people on an AC eating schedule. The sensation of feeling cool or cold occurs due to a combination of changes. Digesting food takes work, and that work of the stomach and intestines churning and squishing back and forth creates heat. Researchers refer to this heat produced by digestion as the thermic effect of food. The less processed the food is, the more squishing and churning it takes to digest. Less processed foods take more of your body's energy for processing after you've eaten them, so high-fiber, whole-grain meals may produce more of a heat flush sensation than refined, quickly absorbed foods. Putting more energy into digestion means that less fuel is available for your body to store. The thermic effect of food is a good reason to choose whole wheat bread over highly processed products like white bread. The white bread, like other processed foods, is essentially predigested and requires very little digestive work.

Another contributor to feeling cold is your heart and its output. The digestive tract can demand a great deal of blood flow from the heart, causing it to beat harder and faster during digestion. Just as you'd feel when exercising any other muscle, the extra work done by your heart creates more heat than your baseline heart rate. The additional heat produced by your heart's extra work is immediately distributed to the rest of your body by blood flow, adding to the thermic effect of food. With your heart beating harder and faster to supply blood to your gut, the flow of blood to your extremities can increase too, bringing the heat from your body to warm your fingers and toes.

The coolness of fasting brings a tradeoff: it means an extra layer of clothing may be needed in the wintertime, and in the summertime, you may be comfortable on days others find uncomfortably warm. You may save some money by setting your air conditioning thermostat a couple of degrees higher than usual.

If you find the coolness of fasting to be a problem at work and you can't compensate by wearing another layer, you may prefer to use an early window so the thermic effect of food can help keep you warm during your workday.

FAQ (FREQUENTLY ASKED QUESTIONS)

Isn't eating late in the evening bad for my health?

Eating late in the day is not a good idea if you eat breakfast, lunch, and dinner, because it takes away the last opportunity your body has to reach a long interval of low insulin levels. Low insulin levels are good for burning fat rather than storing it. If you're fasting most of the day, it doesn't matter whether you eat early or late—your body still gets the opportunity to burn fat.

I was losing fat steadily for a while, but now it hasn't changed in the last few weeks. What can I do?

This time of holding steady is called a plateau. Your body has lost some weight and is temporarily holding onto your remaining surplus fat supply. It will eventually let go of more, but you don't have to completely yield to the body's natural timing to get back to losing fat. The following techniques may help you speed up the pace in breaking through the plateau. Once broken, fat is lost at about the same rate as before, and you may reach other plateaus before getting to your goal.

PLATEAU-BREAKING TECHNIQUES:

- For a short time (two weeks or so) increase your exercise by 20 percent or more.

- Consciously cut your calorie intake for about two weeks. Consistently cutting half a serving of one item in your meal can be enough to make a difference.

- Temporarily cut your window duration by an hour or two.

- If you're feeling up to it, extend your fast on one or more occasions by 12 – 24 hours.

- Try a schedule holiday—a day or two off of your AC eating schedule, then return to your usual schedule.

People holding at a plateau have reported having increased hunger just before the weight loss begins, so try to think of increasing hunger as a good thing.

Is a shorter eating window okay?

Yes. The AC eating schedule should be a balance between being as easy as possible while still working. If you find yourself comfortable with a five hour window and want to try a shorter one, or if a shorter window fits your schedule or preferences better than a five-hour window, shortening the window may improve the long-term benefits of your AC eating schedule.

Can my window be a different time from day to day?

Success with a sliding window varies from person to person and schedule to schedule. This is one of the many places where one should start with a fixed schedule, and after achieving a comfortable steady state of fat loss, make changes to tailor your schedule to your preference. If your fat loss stops, go back to what worked. If your fat loss continues, then you have found extra freedom in tailoring your AC eating schedule to your lifestyle.

What can I drink during the fasting period?

Any beverage of zero or negligible calorie content is fine: water, flavored water, seltzer water, club soda, coffee, or tea. Decaf coffee is suggested to reduce the stimulant effects of caffeine. See the "Artificial Sweetener" question below for information on artificially sweetened beverages. Small amounts of lemon or lime juice for flavoring are acceptable. Some herbal teas are coated with sugar or fruit juice. If your herbal tea tastes sweet, it probably has added sugar or fruit juice and is best avoided during the fasting period.

What should I eat?

Decide what you think is the healthiest diet. What would you choose for your child if they would eat anything and everything offered? To me, that looks like this:

· A variety of savory (not sweet) produce with generous amounts of fiber

· A variety of protein sources: fish and eggs, small amounts of other meats, minimizing red meat and processed or preserved meats

· Some nuts or sunflower seeds

· A balance of carbohydrate, fats, and protein with no extremes

· Minimal sweet produce: bananas, apples, pears, grapes, pineapples, melons and sweet corn

Reducing carbohydrates (sugars, pasta, rice, bread, cereals, potatoes) may enhance fat loss

by leveraging an additional effect on appetite correction. Particularly avoid refined sugars: sucrose (table sugar), fructose, high-fructose corn syrup (HFCS), honey, syrup and other sweeteners including concentrated fruit juice.

Can I combine this with low-carb (Atkins, South Beach)?

Yes, an AC eating schedule can be combined with diet programs that specify content, such as a low-carb diet, an ADA (American Diabetes Association) diet for diabetics, etc.

Can I chew sugarless gum or candy?

Sugarless gums and candy often contain calories because they contain sugar alcohols such as sorbitol. Chewing gum, therefore, would not be fasting. Chewing and/or the sweet taste, even without calorie content, may trigger gut activity and increase hunger. If it's important to you to have gum, compare your experience on your AC eating schedule with gum and without gum for a couple of days each way and see if you notice any difference. For candy sweetened with artificial sweeteners, see the artificial sweeteners question. Not only might the chewing action and the taste of sweet flavor in sugarless gum stimulate hunger, the ingredients, specifically sugar alcohols, may cause gut activity, hunger, digestive discomfort, gas and diarrhea.

How can I see quick weight loss with my AC eating schedule?

Appetite correction is not a quick weight loss plan. It's powerful, effective, and sustainable, but it's not quick. A pound per week is the typical sustained average weight loss. Because it's steady, reliable and practical, it has a greater chance of getting you to your goal than a "quick" solution does. For most people, a pound per week is much faster than the rate at which they gained the excess fat.

What about artificial sweeteners?

Artificial sweeteners are acceptable but should be minimized and if possible, skipped entirely. Even though they're artificial, they may trigger insulin release, which can lead to reduced fat burning. They may also stimulate appetite. If their use helps with weight loss, then the overall health balance of good vs. bad tips in favor of using them for the time it takes to lose the fat, but it would be best to get used to drinking beverages without them. If you must use an artificial sweetener, liquid stevia is suggested because stevia is a plant product and the liquid does not have filler carbohydrates.

What about stevia?

Stevia is a natural non-caloric sweetener used around the world. One should not conclude any product is safe simply because it is a plant product—the deadly toxin ricin is also a plant product and completely natural too! Recent toxicity studies have demonstrated no significant threat in using stevia. When hundreds of millions of people have used it thousands of times, as they have with Nutrasweet and Splenda, hidden problems may become evident. Like the artificial sweeteners, the sweet taste may elicit some insulin response or stimulate appetite, so minimizing use would be a wise choice.

What about putting lemon juice in my tea or water?

For most people, it's no problem in small amounts—lemon and lime juice do not have enough calories to have an effect.

I'm hungry all day some days. What can help?

Eating high carbohydrate foods (sugars, pasta, rice, bread, cereal, potatoes) usually leads to more hunger the following day. You may want to trim your carbs. If you're in a plateau period, increased hunger may also mean you're about to start dropping fat again. It may be cause for doing a little happy dance!

During your window, if you ate everything necessary to get all the nutrients you need to survive, wouldn't you be extremely stuffed?

No—consider this: What do we need nutrients (food) for?

1. Fuel — energy to supply bodily functions

2. Structure — spare parts to replace what's used

3. Vitamins and minerals — needed in tiny amounts; included in quality food and can be taken as a supplement if desired.

The human body is very, very good at recycling. When cells or parts of cells grow old, their parts are largely reused. For someone who is not growing, pregnant, or breastfeeding, the need for raw materials (food) to build spare parts is tiny compared to the need for fuel.

We need fuel to keep our bodies going, but if it is stored on our bodies already as fat, then we don't need to be eating it too. For those wanting to lose excess fat, the idea is to "eat" that stored fuel. There is a lot of exaggeration about how much nutrient intake we need to live. Much is due to marketing and some of it is planned to avoid vitamin deficiency. The US recommended dietary allowance (RDA), for example, was developed based on micronutrients, not total calories, when obesity wasn't a problem. It used a 50 percent excess of content to make sure sufficient micronutrients (vitamins, etc.) are available in an average diet for the average person.

Can I eat _____?

People often ask if ultra-low calorie foods such as celery or pickles are permitted during the fast. Eating is an activity that involves both body and brain, so there's more to eating than simply whether the food contains calories. Chewing on a pickle or celery stick may lead to limbic hunger, making fasting more difficult than it would be otherwise. In questionable cases like this, the AC test applies: if you see progress while eating something, then obviously that tweak works for you and you can continue it. If you're not seeing success, your tweak failed the AC test. Many people have asked if they can eat various no-carb foods such as olive oil or protein shakes during the fasting period. Eating anything during the fasting period, even something that does not produce an insulin surge, may impair your progress because eating calories of any sort supplies fuel and you burn what you're consuming instead of what you're trying to burn off your belly or thighs.

However, no two people are alike and what is a problem for others may not be a problem for you.

What works for you is all that matters, so you can try any modification you wish. If your modification works, you keep losing weight. If it doesn't, you stop losing weight. You can always go back to what worked, and all you risk by trying something new is a slow-down or halt in your rate of fat loss. Once you've started on an AC eating schedule using the traditional style (no calorie intake during the fasting period) and see some steady weight loss, you know what works. After that, you can experiment and see what modifications work for you.

If you are considering adding milk, cream, coconut oil or anything else to your morning coffee, remember that what you're adding is fuel, and fuel that you consume with your coffee will be burned instead of fat pulled from your body's fat stores. It's your choice. Which fuel do you want to burn? Something that's coming from a bottle in your fridge, or something that's coming from the fat-fridge of your waist and thighs?

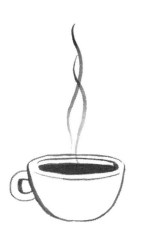

Don't I need to count calories or eat a certain fraction of my total daily energy expenditure (TDEE)?

No, people on an AC eating schedule that's working do not have to count calories or estimate their TDEE. Every non-human animal on the planet that isn't fed by humans maintains an appropriate body fat content without counting calories and without calculating a TDEE. You can do the same, because you have the same kind of intake measurement system in your body as they do. Like all those other animals, your fantastic human body is equipped with an amazingly good appetite center that just needs time and a little help to work. There are some people working on finding their AC lifestyle who use calorie counting as a complementary tool in conjunction with an eating schedule. The combination allows them to see progress. It's okay to count calories. However, needing to count calories indicates that true appetite correction has not yet been achieved.

Won't fasting all day put me in starvation mode?

It won't. It takes at least 48 hours of fasting to activate the body's starvation mode mechanisms. When you're eating according to your appetite every day, you're not in starvation mode. As long as your body has plenty of fuel (fat) to draw on, it's not starving—it's getting all the calories it needs from the breakfasts, lunches, dinners and snacks you ate a long time ago, which you stored in the form of fat. Fat, as mentioned earlier, is nature's refrigerator, and if you have surplus fat, you've done a bit of overstocking of your fat-fridge. Let your body eat all it wants from your fat-fridge. If your body tells you that you don't need to eat more, you can trust it.

What if I skip a day or two? Or go off schedule on the weekends?

Taking a day or two off from your AC eating schedule because of a change in work schedule or social circumstances is not a problem—you won't immediately lose your adaptation. You may experience clock hunger at mealtimes when you resume your AC eating schedule. Some people see progress when they consistently stay on their AC eating schedule on weekdays and relax their schedule on the weekends, but many do not. This is another time when the AC test comes in handy. If you tweak your AC eating schedule by taking weekends off and still see satisfactory progress, then the tweak works for you and you can continue it. If you're not seeing progress, your tweak failed the AC test. Routinely taking weekends off is not recommended as a starting point, but it may work

as an eventual tweak. Skip days don't ruin your AC effort; they only slow your progress a little, and they may help you break through a plateau.

What do I do when I travel across time zones? Which time do I use for my window?

If your travel is only a day or two and you haven't traveled across several time zones, eating according to your home time zone makes sense because your body clock won't adapt that quickly. If you're staying longer than a couple of days, you'll probably do best shifting your window to local time. Different social obligations often come with travel, so you may select a different window altogether. You may decide to take a few skip days while you're on the road and then return to your AC eating schedule when you return home. More than three or four off-schedule days in a row may reduce your adaptation to your AC eating schedule, but restarting will still be easier than it was your first time.

TROUBLESHOOTING AN AC EATING SCHEDULE

If you've been consistently keeping an AC eating schedule for three weeks or more and have not seen at least one pound (0.45 kg) of weight loss, consider making the following adjustments, and remember that any adjustment you make needs at least a three-week trial to show some effect. You may see convincing changes sooner, but allow at least three weeks for changes in your body and appestat to occur before you decide whether to give up on the change you've made.

Although an AC eating schedule works for about 90–95 percent of the people who give it a decent try, there are some people for whom it does not work. If it were clear who those people are, I'd put that in the introduction so no one would waste time on a futile endeavor. So far, no distinguishing characteristics have emerged that predict whose out-of-tune appestats might be most easily corrected using a different tool, or an AC eating schedule plus one or more other tools described in this book.

First, review the basic rule: Consume no calories outside your five-hour window. Make sure that nothing you're drinking during the fasting period contains calories. Some tea has fruit in it or is coated with fruit juice, sugar or honey and sold without an ingredients list. If a drink tastes sweet and you haven't added an artificial sweetener, it's a safe bet it contains a significant number of calories.

If you've given the basic AC eating schedule rule a solid try for at least three weeks after adaptation and you've seen zero weight loss, try these stepwise, not all at once: Most people can eat what they want and see progress. A few people didn't see progress until they combined a low-carb menu with an AC eating schedule, and then they saw good results. You may have a similar experience, particularly if you tend to eat a lot of refined sugar, pasta, rice, breads, cereals or potatoes. Start by avoiding sugary foods like jams, jellies, honey, icing, cakes, sweetened drinks and frosting.

> During your fasting period, you should be eating nothing and drinking nothing that contains calories.

SOME ADDITIONAL STEPS THAT MAY BE HELPFUL:

- Avoid fructose for a couple of weeks, including regular table sugar (which contains fructose), high fructose corn syrup, corn syrup, and high-sugar fruits: apples, bananas, grapes, pears, pineapples, melons and sweet corn (yes, corn is a fruit).

- If you're chewing gum during your fasting period, try going without it. Sugarless gum is not calorie-free. Some people can see progress while chewing gum and some can't, so it's considered a tweak and should be dropped if you're not seeing satisfactory progress.

- Mentally tune in to your appetite. As you're eating, take stock of your hunger. When it has subsided, stop eating and get away from the table and do something else. Some find a little internal dialogue to be helpful. Ask yourself, "Are you hungry?" The answer to that question will be "no" long before you can answer the more commonly asked question "Are you full?" in the same way. Focus on eating until you're no longer hungry, rather then stopping only when you're feeling full (stuffed.)

- If you're eating two meals within your window, try to eat most of your intake in one big meal with a snack as desired afterward.

- Shorten the window to three hours, or even two. You still have time to eat and then eat a little more if you want to.

- It may help to add exercise. Your body will probably increase your appetite to pay for the calories you burn while exercising, but exercise may increase your metabolic rate even when you're not exercising and may help suppress your appetite.

- Add bulk early in your window by eating water-rich foods. Water has no calories, so large volumes of these foods may have a relatively low calorie content. For example, you can break your fast with a big serving of soup, which contains a lot of water. Adding additional water to your break-fast soup can help extend this early, bulky part of your meal. Other foods with high water content (tomatoes, cucumbers, pickles and cooked vegetables such as squash or zucchini) can also help start off your break-fast meal with watery bulk that has flavor, texture and variety.

88

- Timed stepping gives your body a chance to register what you've eaten and may help when an AC eating schedule isn't working. Timed stepping starts with planning a fixed amount of break-fast before your window opens. When your window opens, eat the break-fast meal slowly. When you are done, get away from the food/kitchen/table and remind yourself you'll eat more later if you want to. Set a timer for 30 minutes and get busy doing something else. When the timer goes off, if you're still feeling the need to eat, prepare another "course", eat it slowly, and set the timer again. The 30-minute intervals between courses allow your body to do some digestion and get some sense of the calorie intake you've provided. You'll get plenty to eat and the timed stepping helps avoid any tendency toward binge eating.

- Some foods such as wheat or coffee may have idiosyncratic effects, meaning they affect you differently than most people. Try a three-week holiday from any food or drink that you consume a lot of and see what happens.

- If you're taking any over-the counter medicines or using any supplements, see what happens if you stop taking the product for at least three weeks. Do not stop any prescribed medication without consulting the prescribing physician.

- If nothing else helps, ask your doctor for a thyroid hormone test. Thyroid hormone regulates metabolism, and some of the people who found Fast-5 ineffective found their thyroid hormone level to be low.

SET PLAYS

When you're adapting to your new schedule, there are two concerns you are likely to have. The first concern is that you'll be hungry leading up to the time your eating window opens. You may also wonder if hunger will cause you to stumble in your effort.

The proper approach to these concerns is preparation. A slip is just a slip. It's not on obstacle and nobody expects you to slide into your new schedule with no effort at all. If you slip, try again. Trying again pushes your body to adapt. You can rest assured that most people find adaptation to be much less difficult than they expect it to be. As mentioned before, the real turbulence in adopting the schedule comes from critical friends and family and from social friction, not from hunger.

If adapting to an AC eating schedule were super-easy, a person with surplus fat would be a rare sight. The adaptation does take effort, and it takes a bit of resilience. If you have a plan for what you'll do if you get uncomfortably hungry, you can effectively dispatch both concerns.

The best prevention for somatic hunger is distraction, so if you have a maneuver in mind ahead of time, you can be ready to deal with the turbulence of the transition and deflect whatever hunger you might encounter. Knowing that you're ready to deal with whatever may come boosts your confidence. Confidence leads to an empowered mindset, which makes it less likely that something will knock you off track.

In sports, the planned set of actions for an event that can be anticipated (such as a corner kick in soccer) is called a set play. If you have a set play in mind to defend against hunger, it can be much easier to manage.

YOU CAN SELECT ONE OF THESE AS YOUR SET PLAY FOR HUNGER, OR COME UP WITH YOUR OWN.

- Take a 5-minute walk or other break for distraction.

- Respond verbally or mentally, telling your body that it's not time to eat yet, but that time will come soon.

- Connect with a friend, AC buddy or with an online group so you can check in and share support.

- Keep your preferred no-calorie drink in reserve and drink it as a reward for powering through the hungry moment.

- Brush your teeth (this reminds your body that it's not time to eat).

Support Groups

One more thing…another bit of helpful info you should have for a quick start on your AC journey is the support of others with experience. Please visit the author's website (**BertHerring.com**) for links to the active public and private Facebook and forum alternatives.

**DECIDING NOW MAKES IT EASIER LATER.
WHAT WILL YOUR SET PLAY FOR DEALING WITH HUNGER BE?**

II. DOING

Tool 3: Address the Stress

From the time of the very first animal, there were two threats to survival: lack of food (starvation) and being eaten. These two threats are the most primitive stresses that a creature faces.

To protect against being eaten, animals developed physical defenses (things like turtle shells and porcupine quills) and behavioral defenses (running/jumping, kicks, herding together). An animal that's well equipped to defend itself has little need to feel the primitive stress prompted by the approach of a predator, but what about the other primitive stress—the lack of food?

By the time starvation is affecting an animal, the animal is weak and it's too late to do much about it. The weakened animal is poorly equipped to move around to hunt or gather food and its chances of survival are virtually zero. If an animal

could somehow determine that things weren't going well before the effects of starvation actually set in, then the automatic systems could prepare in advance and the animal would have a better chance of survival. Well, guess what? We're built to survive! Animals—including humans—have stress meters built in to their automatic systems. Your primitive brain core monitors your stress, and as it does in other animals, will prompt you to keep more in reserve if your food supply becomes unreliable.

There's a problem, though. As nice as it is to have a stress meter to help prevent starvation and to alert us to predatory threats, the built-in stress meter developed millions of years ago—before jobs, money and other sources of stress became part of day-to-day human experience. Our built-in stress meters lack the ability to tell the difference between primitive and modern stresses. When stress of any kind climbs, our automatic systems kick in and interpret this as a need to prepare for the impending unavailability of food. The brain-core autopilot has only one response: Eat more when food is available so the excess can be stored as fat.

For most of us, food scarcity is not one of the problems we face, so eating more food and storing more fat only add to our problems and may even add to the stress. For some people, the stress-eat-stress feedback can turn into a vicious cycle.

What happens when financial stress rises? The stress meter says, "Eat more! Store more fat!" And when relationship stress rises? The stress meter says, "Eat more! Store more fat!" And when your job piles on work on a tight deadline? Your stress meter has no idea what that means. If there's stress, there's only one thing to do about it: "Eat more! Store more fat!"

The relationship between stress and fat gain is well known. One of the key stress-related hormones, cortisol, can decrease inflammation. Because of its anti-inflammatory effect, cortisol is often used to treat severe inflammation in someone who has an autoimmune disease like arthritis or other inflammatory disease such as asthma. One side effect of such treatment is predictable: increased appetite, which leads to storing more fat.

Because the stress meter is blind to the various causes of modern day stress and interprets all stress as good reason to increase appetite and store fat, it's important to address stress. While the specifics of all techniques of stress reduction are beyond the scope of this book, you can work with a few of the common ones:

1. **Take a stress inventory** so that you're aware of all the stresses you and your body are coping with. The thing that's causing the stress is called the stressor. Childcare and financial responsibilities are common stressors. While taking an inventory, be honest with yourself about the stressors in your life. Which are the biggest stressors in your life? Consider these and note that there are many other possible stressors.

   - Family/home: schedule, housekeeping, yard care, meal preparation, relationships, maintenance
   - Work: sense of meaning, financial security, retirement planning, job performance, relationships, promotion possibilities, alternatives

- School: academic performance, extracurricular activities, relationships, future plans, financial needs

- Self image: How you feel about yourself can supply ridiculous amounts of stress. If you don't like yourself, how can you expect others to like you? You may be trashing relationships without realizing it.

None of these stresses is life-threatening like starvation, but your stress meter still registers them in the same way—it can't tell the difference, and triggers automatic responses as if a frigid, desolate winter famine were imminent. Take a moment to remind yourself that the stresses you list in your stress inventory are not life-threatening and eating more will not provide a survival advantage. Eating less may actually provide some advantage for many people.

What are your stressors?

2. **Address the stress:** See the stress for what it is and see what you can do about it. What's your biggest stressor? Finances? Family? Often the uncertainty around a situation makes it much more stressful than it is when you have listed the details and have created a plan to deal with the individual items on the list.

3. **Manage the stress.** If you can't get rid of the stressor or reduce its impact on your life, try to vent the stress. Techniques for venting stress include meditation, exercise, counseling, yoga, playing (yes, playing! Go out and play, or play a game!), dedicated relaxation time (by yourself or with a friend). Don't forget sex, which can mix exercise, play and dedicated relaxation time. Writing to yourself in a journal or diary, or writing to a friend can also help you relax or compose your thoughts. Try writing on real paper for a nice change. Reading a book just for the fun of it or taking a bath (or both at the same time) may also help.

Managing stress may be easier and more effective if you have the assistance and insights of a professional. If stress is keeping you from your goals, consulting a counselor, coach or mentor may be well worth the investment.

HUMAN STRESS METER

MODERN SOURCES OF STRESS	LOW	MODERATE	HIGH	EXTREME
Workplace Challenges	○	○	●	●
Financial Constraints	○	○	●	●
Relationships	○	○	●	●
Parental Responsibilites	○	○	●	●
Other	○	○	●	●

OVERALL STRESS LEVEL	WHAT YOUR BODY THINKS IS GOING ON	YOUR BODY'S RESPONSE
LOW	Life is good.	Eat what you need and make babies.
MODERATE	A famine is coming.	Eat more and make babies.
HIGH	It's a famine and life is tough.	Eat a lot more and make babies.
EXTREME	There's no food; predators are circling.	Eat all you can; maybe babies can wait.

Tool 4: Activity

BE A MOTIONAL PERSON

Our culture really does suck the life out of us in some ways. We tell kids to sit still, and then wonder why they put on too much fat. It's time to let your wiggly, fidgety inner child out again. Exercise is essential for good health. Even if you can only do a little, do it regularly. Make it part of your daily or weekly routine. Exercise by itself is not a good way to compensate for overeating, because you have to walk a mile to burn off every 100 excess calories ingested. That means it takes 20 minutes of dedicated activity just to fix a couple of bites of overeating. Getting the appestat working right so that overeating doesn't happen can save you a lot of time and effort.

Even though exercise is a fairly ineffective way to lose fat, it does help get your appestat working properly. It doesn't take much exercise to

see some effect on your appestat, and the exercise can be either dedicated (meaning you set aside time just for exercise) or ambient exercise you do while engaged in day-to-day activities (examples: fluttering fingers, squeezing a stress ball, lifting your heels at your desk, balancing, shoulder shrugs, standing on tiptoe, or standing while working). Twenty minutes of dedicated exercise at least three times a week will help. If you can't work that into your schedule, work in what you can—that's the ambient exercise. Parking in a distant parking spot or taking the stairs up a floor are easy and convenient ways to add ambient exercise to your life, and every little bit helps. Don't fool yourself into thinking the exercise buys you the freedom to take in more calories, though—it doesn't, and if you start trying to think through your calorie balance, you'll be wrong most of the time. Get all the activity in that you can and let your appestat do the calculations.

If your job has you desk-bound, you're at a serious disadvantage already. Comfortable chairs are the modern curse of office life. If you have the option of a ball chair or other seat or stool that requires you to use some trunk muscles, take it. Put up a sticky note with the word "Action!" on it as a reminder to keep some part of your body in motion. Your action can be as subtle as lifting one foot off the floor a millimeter, then the other. Tense, relax, tense relax, back and forth. You can work your other muscles too, just as you sit. Fidget like a first grader. Lift your left knee a tiny bit, then lift the right. Lean your head to one side, then the other, then front-to-back. Stand as much as you can, easing your heels off the ground a bit, then up to tip-toe and back down. Wiggle your toes, then move up with the motion, tensing then relaxing each muscle group: first your calf muscles, then thighs, hips, butt, trunk and arms, then back down again. Walk up a flight of stairs on your way

Action!

to the restroom. Walk at breaks and lunchtime.

Make activity part of your appetite correcting lifestyle. Whether it's dedicated exercise or an increase in ambient activity, exercise can't be just a temporary thing. Your body needs the activity to signal the muscle cells that they're still needed. If you don't use them, you'll lose them! Activity helps your appestat do the math correctly when it's calculating how many calories it's going to demand that you eat.

If you're intimidated by the thought of exercise, start small. Whenever you find yourself standing, turn it into ambient activity. Stand on one foot for 30 seconds, then stand on the other for another 30 seconds. You don't have to look like a flamingo with one foot high off the floor—lifting one foot a few millimeters will do, just enough so you have to balance on the other foot. You can also rest one foot on the other or position it behind the opposite calf or ankle. Whether you do this while brushing your teeth, standing in line or waiting for a train doesn't matter—it all works the same way. Your body will automatically tense and relax some of your largest leg and trunk muscles to maintain your balance. Once you're doing that routinely, add something different, such as leaning forward while balancing or maybe one squat in the morning while you brush your teeth. Then two. Then three, up to ten. You don't have to break a sweat to get an effective increase in activity. The more you do, and the more often you put your body in motion, the easier it gets. The more smoothly you can integrate your ambient activity into your schedule, the more likely it is that you'll keep doing that activity. When you become a motional person, you can't stand to stand (or sit) still.

NON-SEDENTARY ENTERTAINMENT:

Since the average American's appetite set point is only off by about 20 calories per day, small things done frequently can make a difference. Doing something—anything—during your screen time (computer, TV, video time) and other sedentary hours can help correct your appetite. Standing while watching + doing is even better than sitting + doing. Not only does the activity keep your muscles in motion so they burn some calories, it keeps your hands busy so you're not grabbing chips at the first commercial.

Activities you can combine with screen time (you can also do any of these instead of screen time and expect even more progress)

- Knitting, carving, woodworking, sewing

- Drawing, doodling or painting

- Practicing a musical instrument

- Writing (on a computer, tablet or paper—if you like getting real letters, write one!)

- Preparing meals for the coming week (chopping vegetables, washing dishes)

- Ironing or folding laundry

- Playing a game or working on a jigsaw puzzle (remember those?)

- Reading a book/magazine/news story (it may be sedentary, but it's more effort than watching TV)

What other activities can you do while watching a screen? Is there a lamp to be fixed? Furniture to be refinished?

corn and eat salads instead of smoothies.

applesauce. Eat strawberries, not s

creamed corn and eat salads instead of smoothies.

ples, not applesauce. Eat strawberries, not strawberry pr

instead of creamed corn and eat salads instead of smoothi

ritas. Eat apples, not applesauce. Eat strawberries, not str

the cob instead of creamed corn and eat salads instead o

margaritas. Eat apples, not applesauce. Eat strawberries

corn on the cob instead of creamed corn and eat salads i

martinis, not margaritas. Eat apples, not applesauce. Eat

preserves. Eat corn on the cob instead of creamed corn a

hies. Drink martinis, not margaritas. Eat apples, not apple

rawberry preserves. Eat corn on the cob instead of cream

d of smoothies. Drink martinis, not margaritas. Eat apples

not strawberry preserves. Eat corn on the cob inste

Drink martinis, not margaritas.

orn on the

II. DOING

Tool 5: Be the Wild Mustang

The human body (including yours) is a fantastic machine with incredible capability and resilience. If you had lived in the paleolithic times of 10,000 years ago, or even in the pre-industrial times of 300 years ago, it's unlikely you'd have had surplus fat because getting food, preparing it and living in general took a lot more work. The human body has not had time to adapt to our modern way of life with its low physical demands, effortless food availability and energy-dense foods. Modern foods are acquired for us through mechanical farming and delivery, then pre-digested through various methods. Look at all the words we have to describe preparing food—cooking, dicing, slicing, baking, blanching, braising, boiling, chopping, blending, sautéeing, shelling, husking, canning, roasting, frying, and milling, to name a few. Each method is just a different method of predigestion, and every step of predigestion tips the calorie balance toward fat storage by reducing the energy expenditure required for meal acquisition, preparation, digestion and absorption. When the predigestion step is performed by a machine (for example, a food processor), instead of our muscles (as in chopping), it tips the calorie balance even more strongly in favor of fat storage.

Your body is the winner of a survival contest demanding high physical abilities where food acquisition was challenging, competition was high and survival required digestion of mostly uncooked and unprocessed foods with little of the calorie-dense foods and quickly-digested sugars that are abundant now. The extraordinary human body—a combination of mechanical resilience, incredible dexterity and a remarkably adaptive brain—can outcompete all other species while fending off diseases and parasites.

Unfortunately, our culture has shoved your mustang body into a carousel horse existence with a cotton candy diet.

Here's an example:

A peanut butter and jelly sandwich has about two tablespoons of peanut butter on it, which is about 190 calories. Let's ignore the bread and the jelly for the moment and just look at the peanut butter.

It took a couple of handfuls of shelled peanuts to make the peanut butter, about 25 peanuts for each tablespoon. It would take a person at least an hour to collect that many peanuts in the wild and another 30 minutes to shell them, so altogether the energy cost of preparing the peanuts, not including roasting them, would be about 150 calories. A person picking peanuts and then shelling and eating them would barely do better than break-even on the calorie balance because more than half of the energy consumed would go into replacing the energy cost of collection and preparation.

A person eating peanuts from a jar can easily consume three handfuls in less than five minutes—spending virtually no calories while consuming over 500 calories' worth of peanuts. The good news is that chewing and digesting the peanuts still takes some work. Whole peanuts, as many people have seen by way of convincing evidence in the toilet, are rarely fully digested, so only a fraction of the calories are extracted—at best, about two thirds, and in many cases, less.

Now, look at the peanut butter again. One sandwich's worth—about two tablespoons or 30 cc—contains the same stuff as whole peanuts, but it's finely ground to that creamy texture kids love. Grinding the peanuts to peanut butter is pre-digesting them. The peanuts in peanut butter are ground into bits that are so fine that we can't see the individual pieces. No chewing is required to squish them to smaller bits, and what bits remain are so fine that they are ideal targets for digestive juices and enzymes. Our bodies can extract virtually all of the calories from peanut butter—all of the energy winds up stored in our bodies, much of it as fat. Nothing escapes digestion and absorption to wind up in the toilet. Add the calories from the pre-digested wheat in the bread and the predigested and sweetened ground fruit in the jelly and what does that make the sandwich? It's a predigested, fully absorbable calorie bomb.

As another example, consider orange juice. An eight-ounce glass of orange juice is the predigested serving of three to eight oranges. Can you imagine sitting down with eight oranges and eating every one?

That'd take a while, and it would take some energy to do all that peeling and eating. The juice takes no time or energy to peel and has no structure remaining that could slow digestion. The juice may even have the pulp removed so there's nothing left but rapidly absorbable, high-sugar fuel. If your diet consists mostly of predigested foods, your menu is looking a lot like reverse liposuction—injecting more fat into your fat.

As if that were not bad enough, while they're grinding things beyond recognition, manufacturers often add sugar and salt to sweeten the deal. In the name of convenience, we've found ways to guzzle thousands of calories without ever having to take a real bite. Milkshakes, lattes, and alcohol-containing specials like margaritas and daiquiris make it very tasty and convenient to guzzle a thousand calories in just a few minutes.

Predigestion by grinding used to be reserved for baby food and puréed meals in nursing homes. In the name of convenience, most foods are now predigested in some way (yes, that includes smoothies).

Instead of going for smoothies and other pasty renditions of food, try to stick with foods that look like the original item.

> Take your mustang body off the carousel and feed it some "wild" food—food that takes some effort to eat.

If you're going for apples, eat apples, not applesauce. Eat strawberries, not strawberry preserves. Eat corn on the cob instead of creamed corn and eat salads instead of smoothies. Drink martinis, not margaritas. I'm kidding, but only a little bit. You can avoid a lot of calorie bombs by choosing your drink carefully. A martini has about 160 calories; a frozen margarita with the same amount of alcohol has about 500. Both drinks deliver quickly absorbed calories, but the martini is likely to be sipped and the margarita slurped.

Stop peeling your carrots and eat the whole thing.

Eat broccoli and cauliflower raw.

Leftover broccoli stems can be sliced for the start of a hearty vegetable soup.

If you want to eat nuts, buy them in the shell and shell them yourself. They're likely just as expensive in the shell as shelled, so avoiding pre-digestion is no bargain. Nuts in the shell may be a little harder to find, so you might even experience a brief period of foraging to find them. It's more effort, but your goal body is worth the premium, isn't it? Serve shrimp in the shell rather than the shelled, deveined kind. Ice cream is preferable to a milkshake—it may have a relatively high calorie content, but at least you can't literally pour the calories into your mouth. Just to be clear, though, there's no fiber to break down in either, so both will be completely and quickly absorbed.

Predigested foods lure us with convenience and fill most of the grocery store. Milk, for example, is a mother cow's way of predigesting food for her calf so it can get the energy it needs to grow quickly. What would be left in grocery stores if you removed the predigested foods, including bread, pasta, cereal, crackers, cookies, dairy and juice? What's left is produce, canned and frozen vegetables, dried beans, meat, fish, and depending on where you live, maybe some wine, beer and liquor. It sounds a lot like a paleo diet, doesn't it? You don't have to go back in time, though. Choose foods that take some effort to prepare, eat and digest.

SUMMARY OF THE WILD MUSTANG APPESTAT CORRECTION TOOL:

- Convenience and processing of foods leads to rapid eating and complete absorption.

- Respect foods that require some preparation time.

- Enlist family to help with preparation.

- Avoid packaged foods (boxes or bags).

- Don't cook what you can eat raw.

- Slower eating and absorption can help correct appetite.

Tool 6: Meal Composition

More than ever before, recent studies have shown that we are what we eat. For example, a 2011 study showed that rice microRNA (a cousin of DNA) was absorbed intact by mice from their food. The microRNA was interacting with protein synthesis in the mouse tissues. Before studies like these, it was assumed to be impossible for intact microRNA strands to survive digestion and be absorbed from the gut. It's a controversial finding, so more research is underway.

DIET SODAS

Diet sodas, which were listed as acceptable beverage alternatives in the Fast-5 book, are no longer recommended because evidence indicating that artificial sweeteners can fool the gut's equivalent of taste buds (sugar sensors) has accumulated. The misinformation coming from the gut can, in turn, mislead the appetite center. Diet drinks may still be a reasonable tool to help you adapt, so use your judgment in their use. If you start an AC eating schedule and don't see satisfactory progress while drinking diet sodas, please give it a try without them.

STEVIA

Stevia is a natural sweetener that may have the same appetite center-fooling effect that artificial sweeteners do, so while it is acceptable during the fasting period, use as little as possible. Use of the liquid version is preferable to avoid the dextrose and dextrin added to the powdered product as fillers. Growing the stevia plant and crushing a few leaves into your drink is a convenient, natural alternative.

SAVORY OVER SWEET

You won't find the terms "fruit and vegetables" used here because many fruits (peppers, tomatoes, cucumbers, squash, okra) are thought of as vegetables. Most very sweet plants such as apples, bananas, pears, pineapples and watermelon, are fruits. Sugar cane and sugar beets are very sweet too, but neither is a fruit. Most fruit juices, especially commercially produced ones, are essentially sugar water with no redeeming health value.

High-glycemic index foods such as sugars, pasta, rice, bread, cereal and potatoes (S-P-R-B-C-P, which you can remember as "super-BCP") are quickly digested and quickly absorbed. Foods from this group have been reported to increase appetite and somatic hunger the day after they are eaten.

Reducing the amount of SPRBCP foods that you consume by substituting savory plants and mushrooms for them will help your appestat work properly. You do not have to eliminate SPRBCPs entirely from your intake to see a positive effect on your appestat. SPRBCPs comprise such a large part of the typical Western dietary intake that a substantial, sustained reduction in SPRBCP foods can be made without eliminating them entirely, helping to correct your appetite without a totalitarian, austere sacrifice.

SOUPS

Broth-based soups are one of the most satisfying, savory low-calorie meals around because they have lots of flavor, but most of the volume is water. Factory- and restaurant-made cream-based soups can be salt-enhanced calorie bombs, so careful selection is necessary to find the best combination of flavor and calorie content. Most commercially prepared soups add excessive amounts of salt. Salt's not such a bad thing, and our bodies need some of it, but if you'd rather taste the soup ingredients and not just salt, consider making your own soup or mixing a regular soup with one that is either low-salt or no-salt. Soup can make boring plants into a fulfilling meal, and it's easy to store and reheat.

SALAD

Salad is the centerpiece of healthy meals, and the more variety you put into it, the healthier it can be. You can rotate through a variety of greens and toppings to keep it fresh. Most retail salad dressings have added sugar, so consider making your own with oil, vinegar and spices. Mixing salsa with sour cream or yogurt makes tasty dressings, too. As a shortcut to trial and error, you might try searching for a recipe for your favorite dressing online and cut down or leave out the sugar. On the next page, there's a list of ingredients to consider to add some variety to your salad; if you need more variety, browse the thousands of salad recipe ideas available online.

AVOID:

Avoid sugary drinks, juices and minimize intake of the plants highest in sugars (apples, bananas, grapes, melons, pears, pineapples). Ounce for ounce, apple juice has more sugar in it than cola drinks and has no redeeming nutritional value. It's so devoid of nutritional content that manufacturers often add vitamin C just so there's something good to shout about on the label.

ADD NEW THINGS

More and more evidence is accumulating that not only do we digest food into little bits and absorb those bits; those little bits can be absorbed in large enough pieces to affect our bodies in important ways. In a pregnant woman, these absorbed bits can even pass through the placenta to the fetus and affect development. Scientists are finding that not only are you what you eat, but what you eat can influence your health in ways that would not have been considered plausible twenty years ago. Since bacteria in your gut can also influence your

digestion and health, science is taking a fresh look at the huge potential that dietary intake has to improve human health.

Because of this potential to improve human health (including yours), it's not only important to make traditionally healthy choices, but also to maintain a variety in your food intake. You know all those vegetables you pass by in the produce section of the grocery store with weird names like tomatillos and jicama? Have you ever had a persimmon, quince or pomegranate? Next time you're in the store, buy one and search online for a recipe. You may be pleasantly surprised with the new flavor choice and broaden your palette of healthy choices.

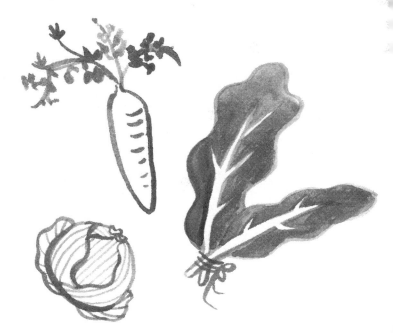

LEAFY GREENS:

- Cabbage
- Cilantro
- Endive
- Lettuce
  (Iceberg, Romaine, Leaf)
- Kale

- Parsley
- Radicchio
  (it's not green, but it's leafy)
- Spinach
- Swiss chard

ADD VARIETY WITH TOPPINGS:

- Alfalfa sprouts
- Almond slivers
- Artichoke
- Avocado
- Bean sprouts
- Beets
- Broccoli
- Carrot strips
- Cauliflower
- Celery
- Chickpeas
- Chives
- Cranberries (unsweetened)
- Cucumber
- Garlic

- Mushrooms
- Olives
- Onions
- Pecans
- Pine nuts
- Pepper slices and slivers
- Radishes
- Scallions (green onion)
- Shallots
- Sunflower seeds
- Tofu
- Tomato (cut, grape, cherry)
- Water chestnuts
- Walnuts

FOR THE OMNIVORE/ CARNIVORE:

- Cheese
- Bacon bits
- Eggs
- Ham
- Turkey

II. DOING

Tool 7: Find Your Healthy Tribe

As you become more aware of how much culture influences the way you eat, you can leverage cultural connection to help you in your quest to tune your appestat. Finding a healthy tribe means building connections with people and communities that are not food-centered and are preferably focused on activity. Finding a healthy tribe doesn't mean you have to give up current friendships, and it doesn't mean you have to meet a lot of new people.

Your healthy tribe can be just one person—a buddy who has similar goals and interests. Using online meet-up tools like meetup.com, you can meet people who are both physically active and share your interests. While many groups on meetup.com are focused on networking or food or beverage consumption, you can find groups for walking, running, rowing, kayaking, bicycling, and almost any other activity. As you build relationships with members of these groups, you may see that lean people are culturally and habitually lean. They eat, but they don't focus on eating as a goal, and they will often prioritize activities ahead of eating.

You might feel intimidated if you show up to an event and everyone is lean except you. Don't let that get to you. One of the reasons the members of the group are lean is because they've been in the group or its corresponding activity for a while. Most active people will understand and respect your desire to get lean, and it's likely that many of them have dealt with surplus fat. Instead of being intimidated and retreating from the group, ask for support.

Meetup.com isn't the only place to build your healthy tribe. Look in your neighborhood for walking groups, or start one yourself with neighbors. Look in your parks for structured or pick-up games. Look in your church, temple, or mosque. Look for activities from campus or park cleanups to board and card games to 5K run/walks. The best activities are those where the activity itself does not prevent socializing, since having fun and meeting new friends reinforces the positive attitude of your healthy tribe.

Building a healthy tribe voluntarily creates positive peer pressure. It's a place where progress feels good and no one will scorn your success. The healthy tribe tool can work in many ways to help correct your appetite:

- Increased activity

- Increased social connections

- Positive attitude

- Positive peer pressure

- Encouragement and positive feedback

- Distraction from and replacement of food-centered activities

- Connection to other healthy tribe activities

MY HEALTHY TRIBE GOALS

II. DOING

Tool 8: Portioning

How many times have you heard the words "clean your plate?" The drive to leave no waste on the dinner plate is very strong in developed countries. After all, if we leave uneaten food on our plates, we are compelled to think of starving children around the world who would be happy to have it. Does eating beyond our own satiety help those kids? No, but it hurts us by contributing to our overeating.

Portion control (portioning) can be a very powerful tool to overcome a somewhat entrenched cultural mindset that threatens to undermine our appestat correction efforts. If you start with a smaller plate or portion, there's less waste. You may clean your plate, and then get some more if you're really hungry. If you're not truly hungry, chances are you won't bother to make another trip

for a refill. Vendors of all sorts use portion control because they know it works. They'd rather dole out small portions and have you come back for refills because they know you get tired of making trips back and forth. Instead of fetching another refill on ketchup, you keep wiping up the same thin streak of ketchup with your french fries. Less waste means less waist!

Three convenient ways of implementing portion control include: using a smaller dish, using a kitchen scale or bite counting.

Portion control can work with unlimited refills, but as you define your AC lifestyle, you may want to set yourself a limit on refills or limit yourself to one fill of the right-sized plate.

Applying portion control is simple. When you eat, choose a much smaller container than you'd

Actual size of a 7-inch plate

ordinarily use. Serve your meal on a small plate. Have any snacks that you want in a small bowl (or custard cup or ramekin). For example, if you're going to have chips or popcorn, serve yourself a small bowl of the snack rather than eating out of the bag, box, or a large bowl. Think about how you eat popcorn—do you empty the container no matter what size it is? When applying portion control, you can have more when you want it, but you can only have your smaller dish full at a time. To get more, you have to decide it's worth another trip, and the number of refills you take provides a conscious reminder of how much you're eating.

Portioning can also remind you to take the time to savor the taste rather than shoveling mass quantities down your throat. It's the taste that's to be enjoyed, not filling your belly to capacity. You might be surprised at how much of a difference portion management makes.

A good size of plate to use is about seven inches (18 cm) across. A typical modern dinner plate is about 10.5 inches (27 cm), but it holds 86.5 square inches (593 cm^2). That means the 10.5 inch plate has more than twice as much surface for holding food as a seven-inch plate (38.5 square inches, 254 cm^2) does. If you pile on food, the difference gets even bigger, because you can pile stuff higher on the bigger plate. A 7-inch plate will hold about 8 oz. (227 g) of penne pasta. On a 10-inch plate, you can pile on 30 oz. (850 g)—more than three times as much! That means you can fill the 7-inch plate, get a second helping and still not match the single serving on the larger plate.

Instead of using smaller dishes, you can also use a kitchen scale to limit your servings to a fixed amount, such as eight ounces (250 g).

Portion control isn't a trick to fool yourself into restricting the amount that you eat. It's a tool that helps you stretch out your consumption and provides tangible ways for you to actively tune in to your sense of satiety and your appestat, so that you eat only until you are no longer hungry. Portion control helps you adjust your eating habits by creating more occasions during the meal when you can ask yourself if you're still hungry. That means you have more opportunities to stop eating when you're no longer hungry, rather than stopping only when your stomach is uncomfortably full. Portioning your servings also helps avoid overeating by reducing the amount of food on your plate that's in excess of what your appestat tells you that you need. If you can't resist cleaning your plate, the extra amount eaten by clearing your small plate is less than the extra you would have eaten had you used a larger plate.

Sometimes you don't have the right-size plate, cup or bowl, or you don't have a scale. In that situation, place your portions on a larger plate with wide margins between them—separate them as if they'd turn to tasteless goo if they touched each other.

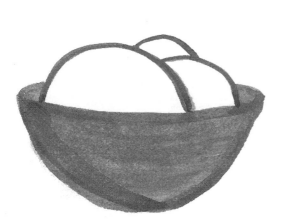

A bowl easily holds 3 scoops of ice cream. Toppings get hidden by the bowl. 164 grams, 360 calories

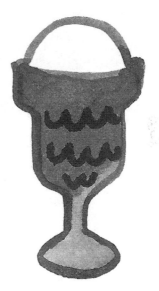

A sundae cup holds only 2 scoops and limits toppings, but keeps them visible. 100 grams, 220 calories

As part of a lifestyle change that encourages savoring flavors (actually getting the most enjoyment out of your eating), there are some other steps you can take as well. Along with changing the size of your serving, you can also change the size of your bite. Instead of a regular dessert spoon, use either a drink mixing spoon, an iced tea spoon with a small bowl or a demitasse spoon. This is the way that many fancy restaurants serve sorbets, so whether it's house brand or Häagen-Dazs, why not enjoy your ice cream with the same fancy flair? You may also want to try substituting a shrimp fork or chopsticks for your regular fork as a reminder to concentrate on taste, not speed or volume.

It may take some adjustment time during which you allow yourself some slips, but eating can become more focused on savoring tastes and indulging in sensory satisfaction and pleasure, and less about eating to the point you're feeling stuffed.

Portioning doesn't apply only to meals; it applies to snacks, too. If you pour yourself a small bowl of chips instead of sitting down with the whole bag, even an out-of-tune appestat can pick up on the fact that you've had plenty by the second or third refill. Fast food can be portioned by ordering on the lighter side at first with the intention of ordering more if you're still hungry after finishing that.

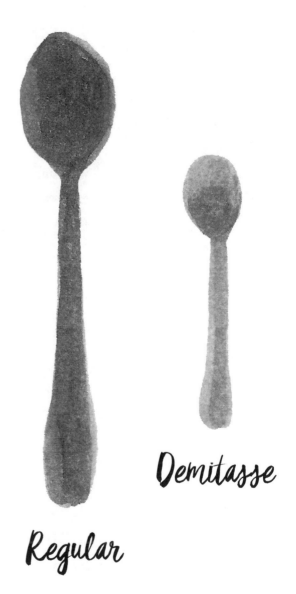

Spooning, AC Style

Demitasse

Regular

Tool 9: Meal Dynamics

Meal dynamics is a way of saying that it's not just what you eat and when you eat that matters; how you eat matters, too! There are a lot of variables in how one eats:

Your pecking order:

Main course, sides then dessert? What about eating dessert first to make sure there's room, rather than stuffing it in on top? It's important to think about how customs guide us, and ask whether it really makes sense. If you know you're going to have dessert, why not have it first (or earlier in your courses) so you can savor it rather than squeezing it in when you're already feeling full?

Pace and duration:

Is the meal more like a tweet or an essay? Is it more reminiscent of frenzied choreography or a slow dance? How long does it take to consume the meal? Does eating carbohydrates first or last matter?

Timing:

If you're eating on an AC eating schedule, do you eat at the beginning of the eating window? The end? Or do you graze through the window on snack-sized portions?

Fast food is called fast because it's quick to pick up. Fast food may be adding to surplus fat in ways that go beyond simply being loaded with calories and engineered to have a compelling, appetite-stimulating taste and mouthfeel. Fast food is fast in another way: not only is it available quickly, but people tend to eat it and digest it quickly with complete absorption. The convenience of a sandwich, French fries and soft drink or milkshake makes it possible to ingest a day's worth of calories in less than ten minutes. With an avalanche of calories tumbling down your throat, your appestat doesn't have time to measure the first bite before you've gobbled down the whole meal. You just paid for the meal, so you eat every bite to get the maximum value. It may not really be the best value, though, because the extra bites stretch your stomach, so it takes more food later to get the same feeling of fullness. Stomach stretch is an important sensation that helps inform you when you've eaten enough, so it pays to avoid "spraining" your stomach by taking in those extra bites. You get your best value by saving the extra bites for later; if that's not practical, discarding the excess is still better than pushing it on your body. Ordering less next time will avoid the waste.

You may have heard your mom or grandmother tell you not to eat so fast, but what harm can there be in eating quickly? It's the same amount of calories, isn't it? How can extending meal duration really help correct your appetite?

There's a limit to the brightness level your eyes can register—a point at which light sources A and B are both so intense that it's impossible to tell whether source A is brighter than source B. Sounds can only get so loud before we become unable to tell which one is louder.

Even though jet engine A is twice as loud as jet engine B, both engines may be so painfully loud sound that we can't tell the difference between jet engine A and jet engine B. The same holds true for odor. There's a point at which one can no longer tell if the intensity of the odor is increasing. The sensors of our bodies are no different than human-made equivalents in having limits to their range. Microphones have a maximum peak of loudness they can transmit. Sounds beyond this range may not break the microphone, but the microphone's ability to relay the signal accurately may be lost as the loudness peaks, and louder sounds no longer generate a stronger signal on the recording.

A camera's digital sensor can be overwhelmed by too much light. A photo that includes a bright light or the sun may be washed out and lack detail unless the light is reduced to fall within the sensor's working range.

The range at which a sensor can provide different responses—from darkest to lightest, from the softest sound to the loudest, from the least detectable amount to the most intense—is called the dynamic range. When the thing that's being recorded becomes so intense that the sensor cannot register a greater signal, the sensor is said to be saturated.

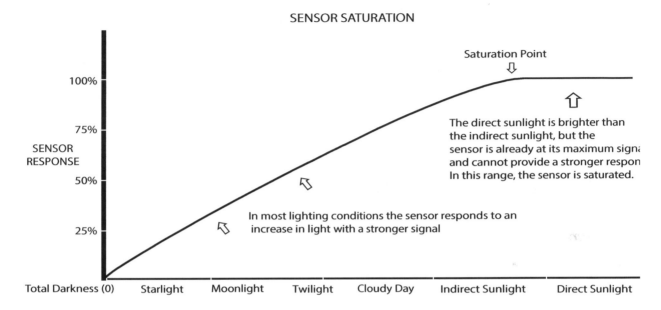

SENSOR SATURATION

Saturation Point

SENSOR RESPONSE

100%

75%

50%

25%

The direct sunlight is brighter than the indirect sunlight, but the sensor is already at its maximum signa and cannot provide a stronger respon In this range, the sensor is saturated.

In most lighting conditions the sensor responds to an increase in light with a stronger signal

Total Darkness (0)   Starlight   Moonlight   Twilight   Cloudy Day   Indirect Sunlight   Direct Sunlight

As mentioned before, humans and all other animals are able to measure calorie intake. No one is yet certain whether the appestat's calorie flow sensor operates using nerves in the stomach and intestine or hormones or both. How the sensor works doesn't really matter when it comes to using it to leverage the appestat by applying tools that you can control. There's no reason to believe that the appestat's calorie intake sensor is different from all other sensors (eyes, ears, nose, microphones, image sensors) in having an upper limit of how much it can measure.

If the appestat's sensor for calories flowing in from the gut is maxed out by a calorie absorption rate of just a few hundred calories per hour, then the saturation of the sensor caused by meals of quickly digested, quickly absorbed calories may blind the appestat to some (perhaps even most) of the calories consumed.

How quickly do you eat? Time yourself and see. You may be surprised. If you're finished in less than 30 minutes, you have a lot of room to expand. Take the time to appreciate the food. Chew it well. Pause between bites. Think about the food—the taste, the texture and the memories it brings to your mind.

APPESTAT SATURATION

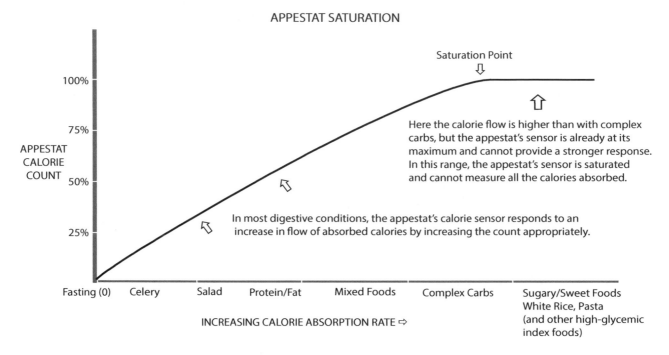

Saturation Point

100%

75%

APPESTAT
CALORIE
COUNT

50%

Here the calorie flow is higher than with complex carbs, but the appestat's sensor is already at its maximum and cannot provide a stronger response. In this range, the appestat's sensor is saturated and cannot measure all the calories absorbed.

25%

In most digestive conditions, the appestat's calorie sensor responds to an increase in flow of absorbed calories by increasing the count appropriately.

Fasting (0)   Celery   Salad   Protein/Fat   Mixed Foods   Complex Carbs   Sugary/Sweet Foods White Rice, Pasta (and other high-glycemic index foods)

INCREASING CALORIE ABSORPTION RATE ⇨

APPESTAT SATURATION: FAST FOOD vs. SLOW FOOD

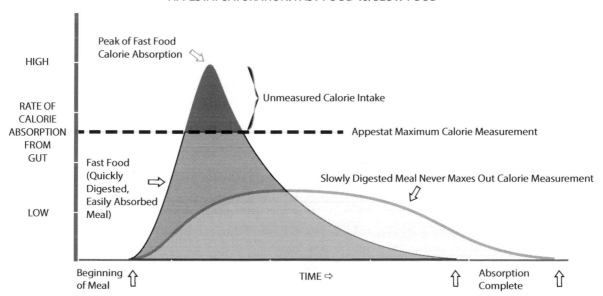

Peak of Fast Food Calorie Absorption

HIGH

Unmeasured Calorie Intake

RATE OF
CALORIE
ABSORPTION
FROM
GUT

Appestat Maximum Calorie Measurement

Fast Food (Quickly Digested, Easily Absorbed Meal)

Slowly Digested Meal Never Maxes Out Calorie Measurement

LOW

Beginning of Meal   TIME ⇨   Absorption Complete

TO USE MEAL DYNAMICS AS A TOOL, YOU:

1. Eat low-calorie, high-volume foods first: Soups and salads are great for this for reasons mentioned in the "Meal Composition" section. Besides soups and salads, you can snack on pickles, cucumbers, celery, carrots, grape tomatoes and other low-calorie foods with high water content instead of concentrated calorie foods like juice, nuts, chips, or rapidly digested foods.

Remember the SuPeR-BCPs

Sugars
Pasta
Rice
Bread
Cereal
Potatoes

2. Take your time! Meals are not a pit stop, where every second shaved off your eating time provides some advantage for your daily race. On the road of life, we really don't want to get to the finish line! Savor the flavors and the company. If you're eating alone, weave in another activity at the same time. Screen time that doesn't require any interaction doesn't count as activity. Read a book, a paper or browse on a computer—any activity that requires you to put the food/fork down now and then can help. If your meal has a time limit (like a lunch hour), stretch out your bites so you're eating at the beginning of the available time and still have bites to take (if you want them) at the end. If you're taking less than half an hour to consume your food, you're not letting your appestat have a chance to register all you've eaten.

Meal dynamics is all about giving your body time—time to eat, time to digest, time to properly measure the amount you've eaten. Even if you're eating fast food, you can help correct your appetite by eating it slowly.

ots, Cab... Iceberg, Kale, Pe... Radishes,
lic, Ginger, Iceberg, Kale, Radicchio, Wa
Peppers, Pickles, Pinenuts, Radicchio, Radishes,
ch, Sunflower Seeds, Swiss Chard, Tofu, Tomatoes, Wa
uash, Arugula, Asparagus, Bok Choy, Cabbage, Collard
eks, Rhubarb, Spaghetti Squash, Watercress, Zucchini, Spro
Sprouts, Almonds, Apples, Artichoke, Avocado, Bean Spro
Cabbage, Carrots, Carrots, Cauliflower, Celery, Chic
ber, Endive, Garlic, Ginger, Iceberg, Kale, Mushrooms, O
Peas, Pecans, Peppers, Pickles, Pinenuts, Radicchio, Ra
lots, Spinach, Sunflower Seeds, Swiss Chard, Tofu, Tor
uts, Acorn Squash, Arugula, Asparagus, Bok Choy, Cabb
ant, Kohlrabi, Leeks, Rhubarb, Spaghetti Squash, Wate
hallots, Alfalfa Sprouts, Almonds, Apples, Artichoke, A
Cabbage, Carrots, Carrots, Cauliflower, O
Garlic, Ginger, Iceberg, Kale, A
Pinenuts,

Tool 10: Making Decisions

Decision making can be difficult when it comes to food, so one way you can help your appestat work better is to keep your food-related decisions away from your appestat's influence. The easiest way to do that is to avoid making food choices when you're eating or hungry. Before you go to the grocery store, make a list of healthy choices and stick to it. Decline the store's free samples. That "one bite" that the store offers in the form of free samples is the store's attempt to leverage your appestat against you. They offer that free bite so that your appestat can take control of your behavior. Instead of seeing scrumptious free samples, see the offer for what it is. The merchant is wielding a tool to push appestat-tampering gremlins inside your head to confuse your appestat so it takes control of your food selections and spending.

If you come home from the grocery store with just what's on your "healthy" list, you've done very well. With only healthy choices in your home, if you overeat, it will be by a few calories of broccoli, peas, pickles or carrots instead of a few hundred calories' worth of donuts, cookies, chips or candy.

With the rising abundance and marketing of sugar and candy, what used to be special occasion treats have become so ordinary that they've lost the fun they used to have. Candy is not an appropriate everyday, on-every-desk treat at any age. Don't let the master marketers persuade you to turn all of your holidays into candy-coated calorie-crunching train wrecks. Concentrate on savory traditional recipes with less sugar instead.

Cookies, candy and cake are entirely appropriate for special occasions, but the key word here is special. You don't have to say goodbye to Halloween treats or birthday cake, and you don't have to eat salad instead of holiday cookies. To help your appestat stay on track, say goodbye to everyday sweets and to celebrating every event with indulgences. When there are holiday treats, scale back from buying bags of miniatures; instead, purchase one or two units of a single-serving version of the treat.

Chocolate is not the problem—it's the sugar and fat that's mixed with it in the candy. Varieties of chocolate are now available with much less sugar, which means more chocolate flavor and less sweetness. It's another opportunity to savor the flavor rather than let your autopilot drive you to gobble up sugar.

> *To help your appestat stay on track, say goodbye to everyday sweets and to celebrating every event with indulgences.*

Even Mars, Inc., the company that makes M&Ms, Snickers and Skittles candies, has expressed support for limiting sugar intake to no more than ten percent of total calories consumed. This may be a move motivated by concerns that Mars Inc. and other candy manufacturers may one day be held liable for diabetes and other illnesses just as tobacco companies have been held liable for lung cancer. The expression of concern is meaningful and can help make your decision-making easier. If Mars Inc. is concerned about the diabetes and health effects of too much sugar, you should be too!

II. DOING

Tool 11: Experiment

Experimenting is an essential tool for developing an AC plan that works as your permanent lifestyle. No one but you has the genes you have. No one but you lives in exactly the same environment in which you live. No one eats exactly what you eat in the way that you eat it at the same time you eat it. Because everyone is unique, no one can tell you exactly what schedule or other AC tools will work best for you. It's up to you to determine your ideal AC plan.

People adopting an AC lifestyle often have questions about which is best, choice A or choice B. Some folks, for example, really don't like coffee without milk or cream, so they wonder whether the added calories will impair their fat loss.

They have:

Choice A: coffee without cream

Choice B: coffee with cream

An experiment compares the two, while keeping everything else the same as much as possible. Many people might try choice A on one day, then choice B the next to compare the two. That won't provide reliable information, because the appestat takes weeks to adjust to changes.

An appropriate test for Choice A vs. B is at least a month of continuous Choice A, followed by a month of Choice B. If fat loss during the Choice B trial month is either no different or better than it was with Choice A, then integrating Choice B into your permanent AC lifestyle makes sense.

Quality of life matters. Depending on the degree of difference and your priorities, drinking coffee with cream may still make sense as part of your permanent AC lifestyle. For example, if your fat loss while drinking coffee with cream (Choice B) was only 90 percent of what it was when drinking coffee without cream (Choice A), the quality of life improvement that drinking coffee with cream offers may make it worth maintaining, even though it provides for slightly slower fat loss than drinking coffee without cream might offer.

To make the most of your experiments, keep your records in a notebook, document file or notes app if you have a smartphone. Record changes that you notice. A change that you experience may or may not be due to the choice you're testing—it could just be a coincidental fluke. It may take a couple of tries to determine whether the change is really connected to the choice you're testing.

When you put something to the test, you may have different results than someone else who tries the same thing. That doesn't mean one of you is wrong and the other right; it means that you're different. That's the point of putting it to the test with your body, your schedule, your environment and your preferences—you find out what works best for you. What works—or doesn't work—for someone else is irrelevant to your AC lifestyle.

AC EXPERIMENT IDEAS

II. DOING

Tool 12: Awareness

You are being used. People with advanced training in psychology and behavior are applying everything they know and decades of experience to get you to eat more so that you'll buy more. They view you as a farm animal in a massive herd—something to be manipulated, corralled, branded and used.

Advertising firms spend millions of dollars on studies designed to carefully determine what compels you to eat more and spend more. This sort of gremlin is a little different from most in that it's not accidental—it works around the clock to exert a deliberate and sustained force pushing to get you to eat more.

Consider what would happen if Americans stopped overeating their average of 20 calories per day. That 20 calories is about a penny's worth of dollar-per-pound dry spaghetti. If you eat that much less every day, that's $3.65 worth in a year. Not such a big deal, right? What happens if every person with surplus fat did the same thing? That's about 233 million people. If all adults in the US with surplus fat were to wave the magic wand mentioned earlier so they stop overeating, the food industry would lose almost a billion dollars per year in revenue.

That's just ceasing the overeating, but the average American has 23 pounds of surplus fat, which is over 80,000 calories' worth of surplus fuel. If all adults with a fat surplus were to start losing fat at a rate sufficient to lose the surplus within a year, they'd each save at least $37 on food that year. That money saved means the food industry would lose $8.6 billion or more in retail sales that year.

If the food industry is not getting the cash, where is it going? It's yours! Yours to save or spend on something else!

With numbers like these, you can see why the emphasis pushed through media channels has been on "eating right" and exercising more rather than eating less. The merchants want you to consume more, and then spend even more on gyms and such so you can burn it off. They don't care a bit that you're paying to burn off the calories that you paid to put into your body.

Why is there no encouragement to avoid consuming the excess calories in the first place? Oh, no, that would put the brakes on both the food and fitness industries' gravy trains!

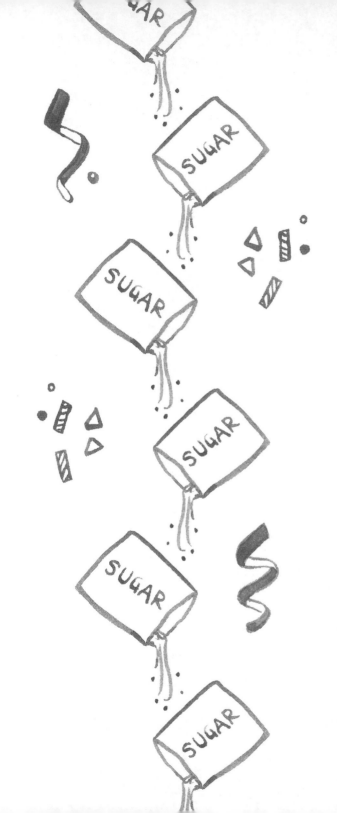

Thus, we see corporations investing heavily in creating appetite gremlins with names like marketing, advertising, psychology, and food science. These gremlins are often very smart and creative people who draw on the latest neuroscience research to find ways to manipulate your decision-making, and they're competing with other very smart and creative people to get you to do something you wouldn't otherwise do. As long as you overeat their product and not the competition's, they've done their job.

There is nobody on your side. No cavalry is coming to your defense, nor any flock of eagles. Government policy handled by agencies like the USDA and FDA is controlled by large corporations. Health and dietetic agencies do not want to cut their own business, so they dare not encourage you to do things that would cut the demand for their professional services. You are alone and under siege. The corporate gremlins maintain a constant barrage of harpoons aimed at your appetite center with the goal of reeling in your consumption and your money using relentless exposures to food ads.

Your best defense against the horde of corporate gremlins is awareness. When the television news/talk show raves about a diet product, is it an advertisement or a news item?

When it comes to media—whether it's television, radio, newspapers or magazines, you are not the customer. You are the product!

The advertisers are the customers, and the media channel is delivering the product, which is your attention, to its customers, the advertisers. The media channels are holding your attention long enough for the advertisers to herd you toward their products and services. If you have doubts about this point of view, follow the money. You may pay unholy prices for cable service, but it is the commercials that pay for programs on the networks. If you watch broadcast TV over the air, it's "free"—free to you, but not free. Advertisers, by buying commercial spots, are paying the networks to make and broadcast programs to hold your attention while the advertisers launch their harpoons at you. Every advertisement is a harpoon intended to penetrate your skull and get its barb into your brain so the advertiser can reel you in. It's not even you they want; all they really want to reel in is your cash, but to get that, they have to reel you in, too.

You may think that giving commercials this much respect is exaggerating their effect—after all, it's just a commercial and we don't have to act on it. A brain study technique known as functional magnetic resonance imaging (fMRI) has enabled researchers to look at the brain's response to commercials. Studies show that food commercials affect far more than the visual cortex. Food commercials also activate the brain's centers for reward and for the mirroring and initiation of eating. Advertisers read these studies and know that instead of using focus groups and surveys, they can design commercials based on fMRI data. In a new specialty called neuromarketing, fMRI and other techniques are used to test commercials to select the one that hits deepest and most profoundly in the brains of their target audience, whether it's kids, adolescents or adults. While scientists and advertisers are still debating the validity of the interpretations and results, the initiative and budget for finding the most effective ways to manipulate your brain and cultivate want are both present in force. Given these techniques, the demonstrated intent and the financial arsenal available to the advertisers, seeing a commercial as a weapon of persuasion and control aimed at your brain is no exaggeration.

In the same way that you can suppress your body's automatic systems and suppress a startle response to a sudden loud noise that you know is coming—a noise that would otherwise make you jump out of your seat—you can also suppress your appestat's susceptibility to advertisements. Use the awareness tool to shield your appestat from the barrage of harpoons. Instead of being one of the many in the herd that gets branded, you can recognize what's happening. You can recognize when the advertisers are trying to manipulate you. When you see an advertisement—which may be more than 200 times in a day—you can announce to yourself, aloud or silently, "they're trying to get me to want something I don't need."

Advertisers don't stop at advertisements. With so much money at stake, they use all the weapons available. In an effort to sell you stuff, corporate PR teams spend their days pushing news stories that make corporations and corporate products look good to the media channels. When one of a network's biggest advertisers suggests a news story about a scientific study that makes the advertiser's product look good, how do you think the network will respond? Will they run the news story or lose millions of dollars in advertising sales to the competing network or channel? Now suppose there's a scientific study that makes the same advertiser's product look bad. Who is working to push that story out to the networks? Nobody!

> # There's no PR team working for the good of the public — that doesn't make any money.

A study that reveals results that are good for the public, but makes no money for a corporation will remain buried in some inaccessible journal and will rarely be brought to the attention of the public through major media channels.

The result of this lopsided arrangement is that the stream of information we call "news" is skewed, pointing out health products and services that can make somebody a buck and ignoring those that don't. Whether the products or services actually do you any good is irrelevant!

Awareness of the barrage of harpoons launched by the gremlin horde allows you to shield your appestat from the onslaught. When you're aware that almost everything you hear and see was pushed at you by someone with something to sell, you can tune most of it out. Think of this with every fast food sign you see, and every restaurant commercial. You'll notice just how dense the barrage is and understand why your appestat might get a bit confused. Examine the ads instead of letting them hammer on your appestat. Ask questions: Why is that ad there? Who paid whom to get this in front of me? Why are they showing that image? Irritate the hell out of the advertising gurus and psychology wonks by refusing to react as they expect. Rebel, misbehave, step out of line, run from the herd! See the siege of gremlins and the harpoons launched at you for what they are: attempts to manipulate you so they can take your money. Deflect them from your appestat with your shield of awareness and eat on your own terms.

ntrol of my eating habits. I d..
at to eat and when to eat. I live a healthy
estyle. I am full of energy. I am open to
ibility. I believe in myself. I am powerfu
m courageous. I can do anything I set my
d to. I inspire myself and others. I can d
is. I will succeed! I am in control of my
ing habits. I decide what to eat and when
eat. I live a healthy lifestyle. I am full
energy. I am open to possibility. I believe
myself. I am powerful. I am courageous.
n do anything I set my mind to. I inspire
myself and others. I can do this. I will
..ed! I a..

II. DOING

Tool 13: Affirmations

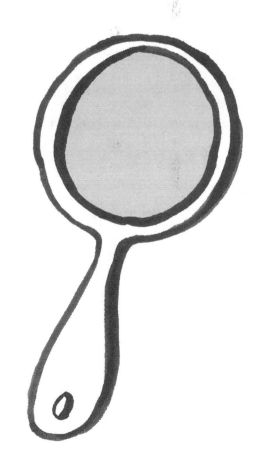

Affirmations are things you tell yourself. They can be said out loud, mentally recited like a mantra, or written. Affirmations can be very effective tools in establishing and maintaining your AC lifestyle. Affirmations are self-coaching. Putting on a coach's hat and giving yourself a pep talk may feel uncomfortable at first, but do yourself a favor and get comfortable with it! Affirmations have been shown to be incredibly effective. It may surprise you to discover how much of a difference talking to yourself can make when it comes to psychologically complex issues like hunger.

Your affirmation can be something you say to yourself in the mirror during your morning bathroom routine, or in the car while commuting, before going to sleep, or during any other regular pause in your day. To work, the affirmation must be repeated regularly.

There are many things you can incorporate into an affirmation. An affirmation centered on appetite correction focuses on managing the appetite drivers that are most challenging to you.

Here are some things you can say to yourself to affirm your ability to push back the appetite drivers. This mindset reinforcement can help you establish and maintain an effective AC lifestyle and keep the gremlins away from your body-vehicle.

You know best where you need affirmations the most. Step outside your mind for a moment and be your own coach. What encouragement would you offer someone in your position? You can do it! You will succeed!

> You and your body are strong.

> You and your body are resilient.

> When you can eat your fill everyday, hunger will not kill you. If hunger comes, it will pass.

> You can go days without food, so a few hours is no problem. It's trivial.

Tool 14: Hybridize

*C*reating the right AC lifestyle for yourself is something only you can do. You're the only one who can say it's just right, and as your life changes, you may find that it's valuable to make changes in your AC lifestyle. One of the things you can do to find your best-fit AC lifestyle is mix some of the successful plans and see what fits your life best. For example, many people have combined their AC eating schedule with low carb (Atkins or South Beach) and have had results that were better than they experienced with either plan by itself. Similarly, the 19/5 AC eating schedule has been hybridized (mixed) with a 5:2 schedule in which two days of each week included a calorie limit. Others have successfully combined it with the 5-bite diet. Please see the resources listed on the following page for more details. The low-carb and 5-bite plans aren't recommended as permanent components in your AC lifestyle, but are worth knowing about if you want to try tweaks as part of a customized, temporary AC plan that may accelerate fat loss.

When you hybridize, it's important to give your body time to adapt and respond. A few days is not enough to see if something is helping or not. Give your body a three- or four-week trial with any hybrid plan, just as you would when testing any other tweaks to see if the new regimen is working for you or not. If you can't keep it up that long, it's not sustainable as a lifestyle. If you don't see steady progress after a few weeks, additional time is unlikely to improve that outcome.

SOME OF THE DIETS
THAT HAVE BEEN SUCCESSFULLY HYBRIDIZED
WITH A 19/5 (FAST-5) AC EATING SCHEDULE:

Dr. Atkins' Diet Revolution by Dr. Robert Atkins

The South Beach Diet by Dr. Arthur Agatston

The Fast Diet by Dr. Mark Mosley and Mimi Spencer

Eat to Live by Dr. Joel Fuhrman

Why Weight Around? by Dr. Alwin Lewis (5-bite diet)

Tool 15: Protect Your Sleep

After thousands of years of pondering sleep, we still don't know what sleep does. We know that we need it, and we know that the effects of stress are more pronounced if we don't get enough of it. Maintaining a schedule that allows for adequate sleep is called good sleep hygiene. If you don't establish good sleep hygiene as part of your AC lifestyle, losing fat will be more challenging. If your sleep is quite poor, losing fat may be impossible. Getting good sleep helps increase your resilience when you're trying to get through the adjustment phase of adopting an AC eating schedule.

What can you do to improve your sleep quality and quantity? The first step is the hardest: get to bed! Getting to bed may be difficult with children, work and distraction, so you have to give it the priority it deserves.

HERE ARE SOME TIPS ON IMPROVING SLEEP:

- Reserve your bed (mostly) for sleeping. Keep screens off or out of your bedroom.

- Give yourself the liberty to sleep later in the morning or to nap when you can to catch up on sleep.

- When you sleep, keep all lights off (no night lights).

- If noise or light that's beyond your control awakens you, try earplugs or a sleep mask.

Feeling sleepy yet?

IF YOU'RE HAVING TROUBLE GETTING TO SLEEP:

- There may be something stressing you that your mind is grappling with in the background. Bring those thoughts to the foreground by taking a stress inventory. Being aware of your stress and its sources will better prepare you to deal with them directly. You may find it helpful to review the Address the Stress tools described earlier in this book.

- Try going without caffeine-containing drinks such as coffee and tea. This is especially challenging on an AC eating schedule, when you may be replacing eating during your fasting window with drinks of tea or coffee. You can try hot water with lemon, or caffeine-free herbal teas for a few days—long enough to see if it helps. If it does help, you'll probably find the switch worthwhile. It's important to note that the labels caffeine-free and decaffeinated are not identical in meaning. Decaffeinated coffee is not necessarily caffeine-free (zero caffeine). "Decaffeinated" means some caffeine has been removed, but not necessarily all of it, and a significant amount may remain.

When you're adopting a new AC lifestyle, sleep may be better or worse at times. It's no cause for worry as it will likely smooth out within a few days as you adapt to the changes you've made.

If you're getting to sleep at a reasonable time and sleeping for at least six hours and still find yourself nodding off or yawning frequently during the day, you may be dealing with a stealthy sleep gremlin. Snoring (either yours or your partner's) can cause repeated partial awakenings that interfere with quality sleep without awakening you enough for you to become fully aware of it. Your partner may already have noticed that you have irregular breathing or unusually loud snoring. Either of those might be a clue that you may have sleep apnea (periods of sleep without breathing due to obstruction of your airway when your body is relaxed). If nobody is around to observe you sleeping, you can record a video of yourself sleeping and then review it to see if you snore loudly or have long pauses between breaths. If you have either problem, a medical sleep evaluation may be appropriate. Correcting a sleep problem will very likely make fat loss easier and improve your life in other ways.

II. DOING

Tool 16: Declutter Your Intake

Be wary of medicines, supplements, vitamins, toxin cleanses and anything else you swallow that's not food.

When you're eating right and treating your body right, you may need less or even none of the above. An AC lifestyle may make many medicines you've been taking unnecessary, including sleep aids, antidepressants, appetite suppressants, high blood pressure medicines and anti-diabetic agents. Do not stop taking any prescribed medicine without first consulting the prescribing physician. Many medicines (such as antihistamines and antidepressants) have been associated with weight gain. If you've consulted your prescribing physician and can safely stop taking the medicines, fat loss may become easier. Oral contraceptives are notorious for adding some pounds, but they're unlikely to interfere with appetite correction and satisfactory fat loss if everything else is working in your favor.

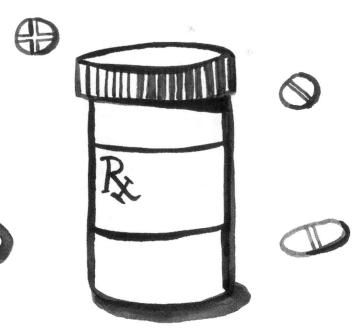

lifetime. Maintenance keeps me from... my goal body. Maintenance is steady-state... ...intenance lets me enjoy life without gain... ...eight. Life is for the living! Maintenance... ...e applying my custom-fit appetite correcti... ...oolkit for the rest of my life. As my lif... ...anges, my maintenance plan can change t... ...ca... really enjoy the work I've done gett... my goal body by keeping up my maintena... ...an. I can tweak my maintenance plan so... ...s my lifestyle. I'm looking forward to liv... ...lean and letting my appetite center count... ...alories for me. Maintenanc...

III. CONCLUSION & RESOURCES

Maintenance

When you reach your goal weight, you will need a maintenance plan. Returning to your old eating habits will make you regain the weight you lost and waste all your work in adapting to and maintaining your AC lifestyle.

You've done the hard part: getting to your goal. Adjusting to steady-state maintenance is something you can fit individually to your lifestyle. You can maintain your AC plan indefinitely. Your appetite will balance your needs.

In the unlikely event that you are continuing to lose weight beyond your desired point, you can adjust by increasing your meal size, cutting back on your fasting days, or lengthening your eating window. You may choose to fast only on weekdays or weekends, if that suits your schedule. Changing back and forth between fasting and non-fasting days is a bit more difficult than keeping a consistent schedule, so tailor your schedule to what works best for you.

...rection for kids starts with offering ...althy choices they prepare for themselve... ...et them decide when they're hungry enoug... ...r stop playing and eat. Kids can help grow... ...hoose and prepare food. Offer whole food... ...tead of packaged items. Avoid sugary foo... ...art a garden. Keep special occasions spec... ...y limiting sweet treats at other occasion... ...elp kids learn to make things from scratc... ...lore old family recipes. Drink water inst... ...soft drinks, sports drinks and fruit juic... ...hoose low-sugar fruits. Air popped popcor... ... cherry tomatoes. Baby...

Appetite Correction for Kids

One of the frequent questions about Fast-5 over the years has been, "Can my kids do this?" Yes, they can, but is it best for them? They can learn how to eat in an innate AC way without a rigid schedule. Children, left to their own choices, will frequently skip breakfast if it means they can sleep later or play instead. If a kid has a last bite to eat at 7 PM and goes to bed at 9 PM, then gets up Saturday morning and gets busy playing, when would this kid get around to eating if a parent or coach didn't push breakfast? Noon? Two in the afternoon? Later? Even a break-fast at noon gives the kid a 17-hour fasting interval. Breaking the fast at 2 pm (1400) creates a 19-hour fast. Kids may benefit from AC with no rigid time constraints.

THE FOLLOWING MAY BE HELPFUL IN CREATING A HEALTHY AC LIFESTYLE FOR YOUR CHILD:

- Your kid won't starve when there's food available, even if the food's not on the kid's favorites list. A kid with surplus fat is not starving.

- Prepare only one meal per day for your child, and let your kid(s) prepare others if and when they want them from components you agree on.

- Keep healthy foods available for your child to prepare and make. Things like savory plants (baby carrots, cherry and grape tomatoes, celery sticks, cucumber slices) can be placed where they are easily accessible at eye level in the refrigerator.

- Offer whole foods, not predigested or packaged ones.

- Let your kid(s) put some work into meal preparation and cleanup.

- Avoid buying sugary foods such as cereals with more than five percent of the calories from sugars. Once you take note of how much sugar is in cereal (up to 30 percent or more), you may opt for oatmeal or eggs for breakfast.

- Avoid celebrating every occasion with sweets. Kids get a year's supply of candy at Halloween and get more at almost every holiday. The average American consumes over 150 pounds of sugars every year. One-third of this total is consumed in the form of soft drinks, sports drinks and fruit juices.

- Buy lower-sugar fruits such as peaches, blueberries, strawberries, nectarines and oranges instead of high-sugar fruits: bananas, grapes, apples, pears, pineapple and melons.

- Kids will be much more interested in eating plants they grow themselves or choose for themselves in a grocery store or farmer's market.

- Concentrate on things that are raw or made from scratch. Most sauces and dressings available in stores have added sugar, corn syrup, fruit juice or other sweetener.

Kid-Friendly, Healthy Choices:

- Cherry and grape tomatoes

- Baby carrots

- Celery sticks

- Unsalted or low-salt nuts

- Cucumber slices

- Radishes

- Raw broccoli with home-made sour cream or yogurt-based dip

- Whole-grain and multi-grain bread

- Brown rice

- Whole-grain pasta

- Cheese (not processed)

- Mushrooms, raw or cooked

- Eggs (hard-boiled or to fix for themselves)

- Green peas

- Green onions (scallions)

- Edamame (soybeans)

- Yogurt

- Soup

- Unsweetened, no trans-fat peanut butter as a treat, in modest amounts. Peanut butter on celery sticks is a classic treat that adds some fiber and bulk.

- Air-popped popcorn (lightly salted and/or buttered; try it with pepper, cinnamon or other spices; let your kid experiment.)

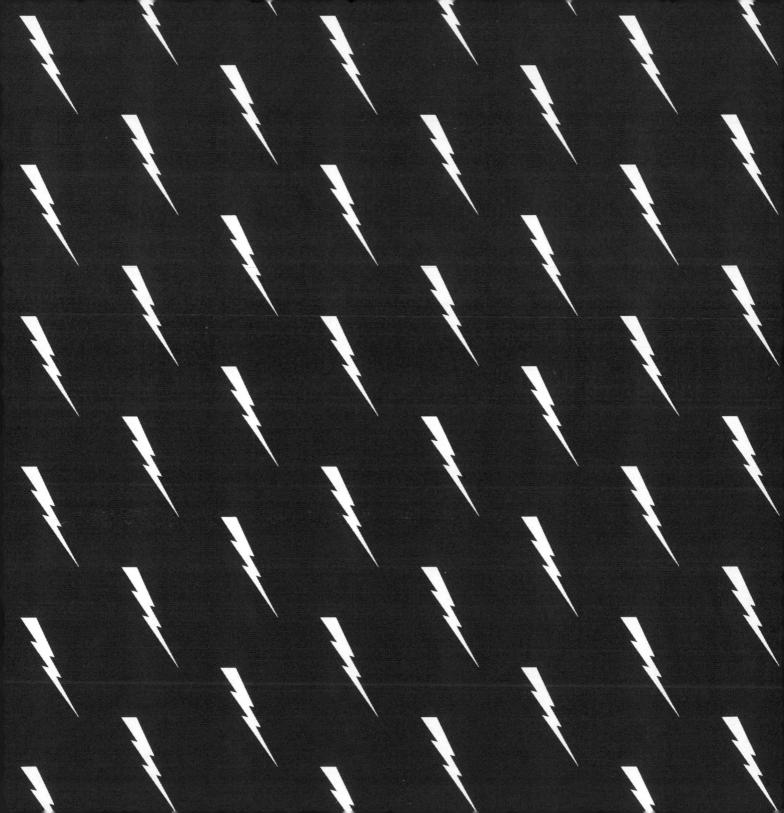

What's AC like?

*n*ow that you've equipped yourself with a set of tools you can choose from, you're poised to start. Let's take a minute to review some fundamentals before you put your toolkit to work:

- Your body is a fantastic machine, capable of amazing resilience, flexibility and adaptation.

- When AC is working, you don't have to hold yourself back from food—you just don't want as much as you used to, and you find better things to do with your time and money than eat. If, after three weeks on an AC plan, you're not noticing a decrease in your appetite, then it's time to try different tools or a bit more stringent use of the ones you selected.

- Along with a reduced appetite, you may see some other signs that things are changing

in your brain. You may want healthier foods. You may feel compelled to start exercising. You may feel like decluttering your home. You may experience some sleep changes. If you have any kind of inflammation like asthma or arthritis, it may bother you less over time. Improvements in inflammatory diseases may take months to notice but may continue improving for months to years.

With AC, there's a tendency to lose inches before pounds—meaning you see the fat go before the scale changes. That's okay, because the weight does eventually go. The inches-before-pounds phenomenon probably occurs because fat that's just under the skin is redistributed into muscles where it can be burned as fuel.

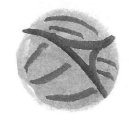

Changes like these may take months to appear, but each time you notice a change, you can savor it as a reassuring reminder that you're doing something very good for your body. It's your reward for putting effort into your AC plan.

There's one last bonus tool to add—the brussels sprouts test. For the brussels sprouts test, buy a bag of frozen baby brussels sprouts and position them on the top or front shelf of your freezer where you can easily see and notice them. These ordinary bite-sized gems can be thawed quickly in a microwave oven. They make a relatively convenient and healthy snack, and can be perked up with salt, pepper or other spices. If you're really hungry, brussels sprouts will sound appealing, or at least tolerable. If you're not hungry enough to eat brussels sprouts, you're not really hungry. Try it out with a package and see if the lowly brussels sprout can remind you to stop browsing the kitchen and do something else when your quest for food springs from boredom, habit or mouth hunger.

The brussels sprouts test helps you become more aware of what part of your eating is true hunger and what is habit, boredom, or appetite-driven behavior.

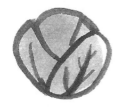

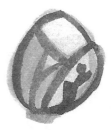

It's time for you to put your AC toolkit to work.

Everyone, including me, has a lot to learn about staying lean in a culture that constantly urges us to consume too much. Please share your thoughts and experiences with me at **BertHerring.com**. While this book began with a starting line, the finish line is not in this book. You keep working with your AC toolkit for life, tweaking your lifestyle along the way so you find an AC lifestyle that fits like your favorite pair of comfortable shoes. The finish line is death and we're in no hurry to get there, so this is not a race. Life is a ride along a scenic route, and I hope it's a pleasant one for you. It will, like any road, have its potholes and low points, but the better your vehicle is running, the easier it is to climb back to the high points, and the longer and more pleasant your ride will be.

GLOSSARY

3MAD

Three-meal-a-day eating schedule (three meals per day)

ACES

See appetite correcting eating schedule

APPESTAT

Nickname for the appetite center's control of food intake

APPETITE CENTER

A primitive part of the brain located near the breathing and temperature control centers that controls appetite, hunger and eating behavior

APPETITE CORRECTING EATING SCHEDULE

Any schedule of eating that enables the appetite center to maintain fat storage and use at healthy, appropriate amounts

APPETITE CORRECTION

A phenomenon occurring with some eating schedules wherein appetite drops in apparent recognition of excessive fat stores, prompting a desire to eat less, sometimes dramatically less

COMPENSATORY OVEREATING

Eating extra (beyond appetite) during the eating window of an AC eating schedule in anticipation of being hungry the following day

BREAK-FAST

The first meal or eating after sleeping, regardless of the time of day; pronounced "brake-fast" to distinguish it from breakfast, the morning meal

INTERMITTENT FASTING (IF)

No formal definition; descriptions of IF range from routinely dropping a single meal from a 3MAD schedule resulting in a 16 - 18 hour overnight fast to a monthly 72-hour or longer monthly fast

NOTES

Made in the USA
Lexington, KY
12 July 2016